DISCOVER A "LIFESPORT" FILLED WITH BENEFITS FOR YOU.

- CYCLING BENEFITS THE HEART—As an aerobic exercise it makes your heart muscle thicker and stronger, increases output, lowers your resting heart rate, and can significantly lower blood pressure.

- CYCLING PROMOTES FAT LOSS—An immediate benefit of this calorie-intensive exercise is that you will build muscle *and lose fat*. You'll discover the power foods to keep your energy high—and a menu to help you lose 10, 50, even 100 or more pounds permanently.

- CYCLING HELPS BACK PROBLEMS—Stationary cycling is often prescribed for chronic back pain; real outdoor cycling keeps you motivated and—like many of the people you will meet in this book —it can help you reduce back pain.

- CYCLING TONES MUSCLES AND REDUCES INJURY—For firm, strong thighs, calves, and buttocks, cycling is superb, safe exercise— and mountain bikes also tone the upper body!

- CYCLING IS GREAT FOR ARTHRITIS SUFFERERS—Without jarring knee, hip, or ankle joints, cycling gives a great workout for people with joint problems.

- CYCLING LIGHTENS THE SOUL—Discover the exhilaration of getting out and cycling—and the feeling of empowerment it gives to those who cannot run or walk with ease. The result is extraordinary stress-reduction, joy, and a feeling of inner peace.

NEW EQUIPMENT MAKES CYCLING EASIER THAN EVER—
AND JAMES C. McCULLAGH
HELPS YOU MAKE IT
THE BEST HEALTH AND FITNESS REGIME FOR YOU!

QUANTITY SALES

Most Dell books are available at special quantity discounts when purchased in bulk by corporations, organizations, or groups. Special imprints, messages, and excerpts can be produced to meet your needs. For more information, write to: Dell Publishing, 1540 Broadway, New York, NY 10036. Attention: Special Markets.

INDIVIDUAL SALES

Are there any Dell books you want but cannot find in your local stores? If so, you can order them directly from us. You can get any Dell book currently in print. For a complete up-to-date listing of our books and information on how to order, write to: Dell Readers Service, Box DR, 1540 Broadway, New York, NY 10036.

C·Y·C·L·I·N·G

for Health, Fitness, and Well-Being

James C. McCullagh

Editor in Chief/Publisher
Mountain Bike Magazine

A DELL TRADE PAPERBACK

A DELL TRADE PAPERBACK

Published by
Dell Publishing
a division of
Bantam Doubleday Dell Publishing Group, Inc.
1540 Broadway
New York, New York 10036

Library of Congress Cataloging in Publication Data

McCullagh, James C.
  Cycling for health, fitness, and well-being / James C. McCullagh.
     p.   cm.
  Includes index.
  ISBN 0-440-50601-8
  1. Cycling. 2. Physical fitness. 3. Cycling—Physiological aspects.
I. Title.
GV1043.7.M35   1995
796.6—dc20   94-36392
                                                            CIP

Printed in the United States of America

Published simultaneously in Canada

June 1995

10 9 8 7 6 5 4 3 2 1

BPR

*This book is dedicated to Robert David Rodale (1930–1990).
He changed the face of cycling in America.*

Acknowledgments

My thanks to the editors and readers of *Bicycling* and *Mountain Bike* magazines. They have taught me so much.

Thanks to Ken Palumbo, Beth Strickland, and Laura Darrow for their help in preparing the manuscript; to my daughter Deirdre and friend Stevie Daniels, for their moral support; and to editor Betsy Bundschuh, for her soft editorial touch.

Contents

ORACLES

I'm writing this during the aftermath of yet another earthquake in California, safe on my farm in eastern Pennsylvania. Soon after the first tremors were picked up by CNN, I received a call from a *Bicycling* magazine reader complaining that he saw no bikes in the auto-infested Los Angeles basin. "Call the mayor, call the governor," he said. Once he had cooled down, he explained he was angry that people don't give the bike its due.

Later I discovered that parts of the quake area were reachable only by bicycle, and cyclists were actually getting to work faster than their road-stalled brothers. No surprise here. The bicycle always comes out during times of emergency, such as the oil crisis of twenty years ago.

I've long had this peculiar habit of collecting photographs of bikes in unusual and sometimes tragic situations, be it the old woman carrying firewood on her bicycle through ravaged Sarajevo or the cyclists charging the tank in Tiananmen Square. These images make the scene even more chilling.

One of my favorite authors, H. G. Wells, wrote, "When I see an adult on a bicycle, I know there is hope for civilization." I feel the same way. In another part of my life I wrestle with the information superhighway, recalling a speech by the chairman of Time-Warner, who said, in a nutshell, "Get aboard or you miss the train." So I'm aboard. I'll likely be chatting with some of you on America Online or exchanging E-mail with you. I'm appropriately digitized.

But there's another road I like to travel, one that is more in keeping

1

with my physiology and psychology. Here I travel at 20 mph, not digital speed. I can touch the heather in the Scottish Highlands, feel the wonder of the holy city of Zagorsk, Russia, and taste a good Bordeaux in France. On this highway, I find fitness, serenity, and joy. I am moving slow enough to reflect on my life and mortality. I touch what's in the air. If I am lucky enough to cycle in Greece, I can almost see the gods and oracles along the roadside.

Don't get me wrong. I like to cycle fast on my Trek 5500, walking through the gears as if I were on holiday. I like to work hard, compete with friends, and crawl into a beer after a stiff Sunday ride. That is as necessary as breathing.

But that's the content of my cycling, not the context. The world I cycle through with its endless surprises, joys, and epiphanies is my real reward, the reason I continue to labor spiritedly year after year. The urchin I met in Carlyle, England, the cyclist with MS I met biking across Ohio, the old school friend I bumped into while enjoying the California redwoods are memories born of welcome. Cycling lets surprises happen. Encounters such as these are what keep me on the cycling highway.

Cathy Dion of Calistoga, California, told me that cycling "is my passion and my cause. It makes me feel alive and free. It is arrival and departure—the journey, the adventure, the life! The changing surroundings, the grass turning green, the birds coming and going, the leaves falling—all these motivate me to continue cycling."

More than one person has told me that cycling brings out the child in him or her. Glorene Cunningham of Highland Park, Illinois, wrote, "Riding gives me a sense of freedom. I feel like a child again. I see things I never notice in a car."

For Michael Tice of Plainwell, Michigan, cycling is indeed an agent of change. "I get better all the time," he wrote. "I learn, I grow, I know, I feel the romance. When I ride, I spend the first 20 minutes sorting out the garbage, all the stress and clutter that's in my mind. Then bang, it's all gone. I am cleansed. The bike, my heart, lungs, and legs are one well-oiled machine in a fluid state. My mind is absolutely empty. I see one big open horizon."

It's not uncommon for cyclists such as Connie Schmucker of Indianapolis, Indiana, to claim, "I don't ride because it's good exercise— that's just the added benefit." Her real reason for cycling is to explore different areas. So far she has ridden in Vermont, Wisconsin, Michigan, Kentucky, Tennessee, Indiana, and Virginia.

Whatever your reason for riding, you can appreciate the sentiments of Chris Etue of St. Marys, Ontario, who can state confidently that she is physiologically younger than hockey teammates more than 20 years younger. She adds, with great satisfaction, "I am aging very well!"

You will also appreciate the view of sixty-year-old Albert Cohen of Davie, Florida, who acknowledges his goal will more likely be the "Tour de Pubs" rather than the Tour de France. He rode a full-blown century (100 miles) a couple of years ago, in under 9 hours, 300th in a field of 300. Though he saw 299 biking buns in front of him, this was a dream come true.

The London *Daily Telegraph* published a photograph feature on cyclists who had recently completed the ride from Land's End, England, to John o' Groat's, Scotland. My friend Paul Wessel and I were among them. The postage-stamp-sized photos of students, housewives, executives, retirees, and vacationing couples from all over the world represented a cross section of society, in more ways than one. We met cyclists who were riding for a charitable cause, to overcome depression, to fulfill a lifelong dream, to mourn a loved one's death, to celebrate a marriage, to bind father to son, mother to daughter, to lose weight, to beat the clock (by racing), to beat the clock (by cycling slowly), to brag about the undertaking, to smell the roses and heather, to get off the information superhighway, to become psychologically centered, to get away from nightmares, to add mileage to a log, to get sober, to meet fellow cyclists, to find a husband or wife, to forget about a husband or wife, to find peace of mind, to become centered on a bike in this "blessed plot, this England," Scotland, and Wales. I took the trip to rediscover the heart of the country I had left behind as a teenager.

From formal and informal interviews I conducted with cyclists who undertook this more than 900-mile jaunt, all had a few things in common. To be sure, all had a reasonable level of fitness before undertaking such a ride. And all took some pleasure in recounting the miles

3

they had chalked up daily. But the overriding imperative seemed to be physiological and psychological health, never stated in precisely those terms, but always present. One cyclist told me the reason she cycled was to be whole again, a remark offered with a straight face and tremendous dignity.

In a way, that remark will become a cornerstone, a leitmotif of the book. You will find a complete and, I hope, interesting repertoire of helpful hints, strategies, training programs, expert tips, insider information, and whatever street talk and intelligence I've picked up during my almost fifteen years as editor and publisher of *Bicycling* and *Mountain Bike* magazines. I'll offer weight loss programs and real life, sensible recipes. I'll take you into the hearts and minds of America's cycling heroes and find advice that is applicable. I'll provide a no-nonsense look at bikes and equipment that will help you sort through all the vagaries of the marketplace, born from a firsthand familiarity and experience. I will offer daily, monthly, and yearly training schedules that will help you reach your goal, be it a 20-, 50-, 100-, or 1,000-mile ride. This book is intended to meet you resolutely and optimistically at your level of need. What I bring to the book is far less important than what you take away.

That is the content of cycling, the necessary and interesting content of a book about cycling for health and fitness. And that's a lot, but not enough. Throughout, I will be obliged to put the brakes on my own enthusiasm because my long experience in hearing from, talking to, and dealing with many thousands of cyclists has convinced me that cycling is the ideal health and fitness activity for man or woman, for any age group, for life.

I never grow tired of saying that I have known individuals who can't walk but who can ride a bike, people with MS and other progressive diseases who find strength and purpose in cycling, men and women who have come back to full health through cycling, those who have rediscovered the "sweet spot" in life on two wheels. It is they who warm my heart and haunt me when I'm moaning. You'll meet many of these everyday heroes throughout the book. They come from all corners.

I am not a medical doctor (my doctorate is in philosophy and literature), and I am not in the business of giving medical advice. I will quote physicians from time to time, when their remarks seem helpful and appropriate. Of course, I recognize the need for heroic medicine. However, this book is meant to be "unheroic," offering the useful and gentle training advice, wrapped in experience and anecdote, that will help you to become, in appropriate ways, your own doctor, trainer, coach, and therapist. I don't say that lightly, since I hold fast to the notion that you can take charge of your own health.

This is by no means a fanciful claim. Americans are too dependent on the medical profession as it is. My approach, my rallying cry, is different. I speak of empowerment—you have the power to change your life, a remark frequently made by the late Bob Rodale, friend and employer, who spent his life reminding millions of Americans of their power within. Bob spoke eloquently of the bicycle as the ideal health vehicle because, among other things, it does no damage along the way. In terms of health, what are Americans most concerned about? The short list would include weight, blood pressure, and cholesterol levels, precisely the items one can monitor without going to a doctor's office. One genuine benefit of the digital revolution is that you can monitor indexes of health from the comfort of your home—or bicycle. You can use a heart rate monitor and a computer to store data on your daily state of health and then "dump" your training and medical information to a disk. Knowing your heart rate is essential to your training program and your health. After all, it's one of the first things the nurse does when you enter the doctor's office. You can really do that yourself. You can monitor your own health. You can tell when you're training too hard or not enough; when to rest or when to ride. Be an active partner with the doctor in monitoring your own health. He or she will salute you.

Lynn La Forte of Murfreesboro, Tennessee, tells me that in addition to riding for the cardiovascular benefits, weight control, and body tone, he rides for stress reduction and self-esteem. "I ride for the soul and heart—love of nature, appreciation of a country ride, sunsets, clear streams, deer, cows giving birth, friendship. My body, soul, mind is refreshed. I feel so much better after a ride—the world is not such a bad place, problems are smaller. I'm happier. It's not hard to ride when you really enjoy it. I stay motivated because I like the way I am since taking up cycling."

While writing this chapter, I've been reading *Revisioning Psychology* (Harper & Row) by James Hillman, a post-Freudian, post-Jungian psychiatrist who, I think, is the most interesting voice in his profession today. He notes that "nearly every individual in the United States of America has been, now is, or will have been in the hands of professional soul care of one kind or another, for shorter or longer periods, for one reason or another."

Hillman is referring, by and large, to psychologists and clinicians, who, as a group, he doesn't consider very fondly. He has written elsewhere that one is equally well off having a beer with a friend than going to a therapist.

The above remarks by Lynn La Forte constitute the kind of self-therapy that Hillman would likely be comfortable with. So without getting too theological, I would offer that to the extent the bicycle takes you beyond the body to a greater appreciation of the sentient world and your relationship with it, you are engaged in a therapy and soul-making, with the latter meaning a reflective perspective on life. You slow down, see things more deeply, and luxuriate "on the edge."

You might think I'm going far afield, but I'm not. I want this book to go beyond how-to strategies, to have texture because life and cycling have texture. I want this book to refresh your body, soul, and mind because in the long run and especially as we close in on a new century, peace of mind and soul will be even more necessary. The how-to advice is hammer and nails, but it's the poetry that nourishes a soul over time.

Perhaps more than any other mass recreation activity, cycling has the capacity to affect positively your body, mind, and soul, perhaps in that order. To be sure, cycling weds you to the machine and if the fit is good, the marriage is better. But cycling puts you in a social setting and in geography, wholesale. Moreover, within this activity and geography you move, sometimes quite fast. Yet you stop and internalize landscapes, reflecting, perhaps, as I did recently on the numerous "veal stations" in and around Lancaster, Pennsylvania, Pennsylvania's Dutch Country. A hut houses the calf and the short chain ensures that the animal won't travel far enough to injure the meat. My observation has little to do with whether or not I eat meat—I do. Rather, it's about seeing, with a "third" eye, the sights and sounds of raucous life we miss from the antiseptic corridors of our daily lives. Or on the information superhighway. When we look at a flower arrangement, as likely as not we'll see the flowers while the Japanese might concentrate on the spaces in between. Cycling permits this visual pause and reordering of vision, thus contributing to our creative health.

I've had the pleasure of appearing on *Today, Good Morning America, 20/20, CBS This Morning, CNN Business News,* and many other nationally televised shows. On these occasions, I often talk about new technology, because products drive the sport. But in my heart I know it's people like you with your interests, your quirks, and your will that represent the backbone of cycling. You know what I mean when I call cycling a *lifesport,* an activity that stays with you through the many stages of life, abilities, and energies. Cycling is democratic and, as tens of thousands of people have told me over the years, "It meets me at my level of need." For Phil Vermeyen of Vista, California, "Cycling makes me a free man; I have not owned a car in 15 years."

Don't get me wrong. This book is about freedom, but mine is not an anti-car message. Fully embracing the ideas in this book, you will enjoy a greater freedom of mobility, a freedom to enjoy space, a freedom to find the beauty in surprise.

Robert Make of Hudson, Wisconsin, has found freedom since he started cycling. Even with no cartilage in one knee, he has lost 40 pounds and managed multiday rides in Montana, Vermont, New Hampshire, Maine, Wisconsin, and California. He has overcome a weight and cartilage problem and found freedom in the new geography he seeks out every year.

This is a do-it-yourself book about improving your fitness, health, mental well-being, and quality of life through cycling. I'll discuss cross-training but cycling will be the centerpiece of my diet. I'll hammer away at the skills needed to make you a better rider. I'll offer a sensible guide to weight loss and add some recipes in the Appendixes for those who want that level of detail. I'll rhapsodize about peaking, going faster, getting stronger and better. I'll discuss road bikes, mountain bikes, and everything in between. I'll walk you through a jungle of products and save you time and money. Unlike most books, this one won't make "buying a bike" a lifetime pursuit. I love the newest bikes and gadgets but know too well the secret is in the legs, lungs, heart, and head.

I've seen enough fit, untutored riders on heavy steel bikes pass the titanium hotshots in pretty-boy Lycra lacking the mettle in the legs. So I'll pay more attention to your legs and heart than your fascination with gadgets. You'll get in the uniform of the day when you're ready. I'm not selling stock in accessory companies. This book, like life, is not about racing. The book is about how to make cycling your lifesport, your joy, your ticket to health. And I trot out every Tom, Jane, and Harry to make my point. These real people with powerful stories made the task of writing a pleasure.

And I believe in putting my money where my mouth is. Once the advice in this book trails off, you'll be able to follow up with me through *Mountain Bike* magazine and America Online. I'm not one of those shadowy authors who disappears into the woodwork after a book is finished. You see, this *lifesport* has been a significant part of my *lifework*, or rather *lifejoy*. I'd like you to be able to echo sentiments I have heard from many other readers in the past: "You have made the difference in my life."

SHOPPING

Most cyclists I know take their bikes very seriously, though not as seriously as an ex-racer friend who actually slept with his, a Schwinn Paramount, a fine racing bike of a decade ago. Richard Lamphier of Elk Rapids, Michigan, goes even further when he asks, rhetorically, "Shouldn't there be a law making it a felony to sell a bike that doesn't fit right? Should there be a minimum construction standard for bicycles? Isn't this a moral or ethical sin? Could the clergy be asked to add an Eleventh Commandment? I think a handful of idiots are having a major effect on thousands of people"—the idiots, I presume, are those selling ill-fitting bikes.

Hyperbole aside, Lamphier would likely receive a chorus of "yeahs" from the 10,000 specialty bike shops in the United States and Canada. Many a specialty shop owner would sympathize with Lamphier, who recounts the following story: "A niece asked me to look at, and possibly make an adjustment to, her ten-speed bike. I found it easier to simply push hard with the palm of my hand and bend the bracket than it was to use a tool to make an adjustment." Surely this is consumer fraud. Well, at least sloppy workmanship and just another reason why so many bikes hang in basements and rest in garages, the eternal lament from the more than 50 million American adults who cycle on a regular basis.

During my tenure at *Bicycling* and *Mountain Bike*, I have ridden, examined, written about, and learned about thousands of bikes. I've been in factories in China, Taiwan, Japan, the United Kingdom, Italy,

France, the United States, and countless other places. I was at the Raleigh Nottingham plant when their bike was a treasure, at countless factories in Japan when that country dominated the world market, in Taiwan when it produced inferior bikes, in China as it learned to manufacture quality bikes for the Western markets, and in U.S. factories (Cannondale, Trek), where some of the best bikes in the world are produced.

I've been in factories where high-end titanium, carbon fiber, and aluminum bikes are made. I've been places that stamp out bikes on an endless production line where little attention is given to quality control. I've seen the same "run" given logos of two, three, or four different manufacturers. Then I've listened to advertisers who try to differentiate the same product.

On more than one occasion, at times risking legal actions, I have with my associates at *Bicycling* magazine fought to keep shoddy products off the market. (That was my nod to *realpolitik,* my reassurance to you that my advice on buying a bike will be straightforward, borne of long experience and tempered by thousands of hours I've spent on factory floors, though this book is not meant to be my revenge for those many bone-chilling hours.)

A BUYER'S MARKET

That said, I've never seen the bike market more vibrant, never seen consumer choices so varied, never seen such a proliferation of quality products to choose from. Translation: In 1995 you will get more bike for your money than at any time in the last twenty years. The same will be true for the rest of the decade. The reason for this is simple: *Competition.* The American marketplace has never been more competitive, which is bad news for the industry but very good news for consumers. However one might complicate the bike, it remains a simple machine. Nineteenth-century inventors might be surprised by mountain bikes and suspension systems, though they would likely find little else surprising. (Come to think of it, the bicycle actually launched the motorcycle industry in the States at the turn of the twentieth century, so the motorcycle features of dual-suspension mountain bikes might come as no surprise after all.) The simplicity of the bicycle and the ease with which a steel-framed bike can be manufactured make it simple for anyone with capital to enter the market. That's why Japanese, Taiwanese, and new Chinese have all but devastated traditional bicycle industries in England, France, Italy, and the United States. And if it wasn't for the inventing and nurturing of the mountain bike industry by a handful of intrepid American designers, U.S. manufacturing would largely be limited to the production of Huffy bicycles in Dayton, Ohio. Schwinn, though now reborn, left the domestic production scene a long time ago.

All this is background music which means, as a bike buyer, you have the pick of the litter. However, it is important for you to know where the litter is conceived, nurtured, and born so when the salesperson smiles in his or her all-knowing way you can be ready and say: "Hey, wasn't that Diamondback mountain bike manufactured at the brand-new China Bicycle Company factory in the Free Trade Zone, a couple of hours from Hong Kong?" And, "Don't the Schwinns over in the far corner come from the same factory? What's the difference between these bikes other than one has Shimano Rapid Fire shifters and the other Grip Shift? Hey, isn't it great the way this upstart Grip Shift took on Japanese Giant Shimano and is making such contributions to our sport?"

Forgive my hyperbole, but I want you to be prepared when you purchase a bike, not for the sake of knowledge per se, but so you can get the lightest, best-fitting, most comfortable, most affordable bike available. Because if your purchase does not meet these criteria, you will not enjoy your purchase, spend time on your bike, or be able to meet your fitness goals. In my opinion, the purchase of a bicycle is as important as the purchase of an automobile because comfort, fit, and positioning have such an impact on your riding. You can get in and drive almost any car. The same can't be said about bikes.

KNOW THE FIELD

Before I get to the nuts and bolts, let me put my biases on the table. In the United States there are two primary distribution systems with other options springing up by the day. About 68 percent of all bikes are sold through Sears, K mart, and other mass merchants. Most of the products are sold for well under $200 through Huffy and Murray, two main suppliers to the chains.

A little over 30 percent of all bikes are sold through specialty bike shops, of which there are 7,000 in the United States. Half of these stores are dedicated to bikes. (Some stores also sell skis, snowboards, scooters, Rollerblades, etc.) A small fraction of bikes are sold through suppliers such as L.L. Bean. Price warehouse stores represent a small but growing part of the market.

My bias is this: If you intend to ride regularly for health and fitness, take an occasional long ride, and want your purchase to have a long life, you are better off buying from a specialty bike shop because the bikes sold there are specced, designed, and built for the fitness and performance rider. No doubt about it, as many of you have reminded me, you can get fit on a department store bike, and if that is your choice and what you can afford, go for it. But by and large, bikes sold through department stores are heavy, not finely machined, and lack the reliable components demanded by fitness riders. These bikes are acceptable for cycling around the neighborhood but not for a serious health and fitness program. Furthermore, few places can match bike warranties, maintenance, and services offered by the specialty bike shops, to be found in every neighborhood in America. So, please take my advice. Get your training off on the right foot. If you're going to buy, replace, or upgrade your bike, go to a specialty bike shop. I don't get a commission but tell them I sent you anyway. Take this statement as an axiom: More people have been turned off to cycling owing to heavy, poor-fitting, unresponsive bikes. Now, just because I recommend going to a specialty bike shop, I don't mean checking your intelligence, wallet, or consumerism at the door. I have a lot of respect for specialty dealers but I well know that their margin and under-capitalization means that the first smiling face you meet inside the door might be the prototypical pimply faced young man who drools over everything new coming out of Shimano factories. I've met this Fred on many occasions. My long-standing habit is to visit bike shops in every community I visit, hundreds a year. If they don't recognize me, they are just as likely to take me down Happy Bike Consumer Lane as you. Days before I wrote this, I had a young fellow tell me his Schwinn line was the only product made in the United States. So buyers beware. Here's how. But first, it might help to know a little about the bike-buying habits of Americans.

Over the years, I've conducted a lot of research on what people buy, when, and how. It should come as no surprise to you or to bike manufacturers that brand loyalty is not what it used to be. Of the 6 million adults (over eighteen) who will buy bikes in the next two years, nearly 5 million are undecided on what brand, another indication that this is a buyer's market. And today's customer is very price-sensitive. Half of those who plan to buy a bike in the next year from a specialty shop will spend less than $350, a reminder to shop personnel that this new cyclist is a significant part of the business.

To be sure, the more knowledgeable a cyclist is, the more likely he or she will say the brand is important. And these people tend to decide before they enter a bike shop, taking advantage of magazines such as *Bicycling* and *Mountain Bike,* advice from friends and family, and "chats" on the various computer networks. Though the specialty shop is the *best* place to buy your bike, you are much better off doing your homework before you enter the store. And you'll want to be armed with some pertinent facts before you take that step.

Remember that, with the exception of Cannondales, most Treks, Raleighs, custom frames, and a few others, most bikes are manufactured overseas, primarily in Taiwan and new China. I do not offer this as a criticism; just an observation. We are in a world economy and the bike is an international product. Through its association with Magic Motorcycles, Cannondale is getting close to producing a truly all-American bike, but that company is in the distant minority. However, I don't think it's altogether an accident that companies such as Cannondale and Trek, who have all or most of their production in the States, frequently sell the bicycle of choice, particularly among the

Enthusiast population. Manufacturers will be quick to add that though these bikes might be manufactured "off shore," they are conceived and designed in the United States—and that is quite true. The irony echoed in many manufacturing quarters is that American bicycle technology, particularly through the good offices of the original Schwinn Bicycle Company, gave Taiwan's Giant, already a brand to be reckoned with in the States, and the China Bicycle Factory a jump start under various arrangements calling for a technical transfer. But again, that is background music. The bike is a rather simple mechanism that can easily be replicated this morning in Mexico, today in China, and tomorrow in India. As a consumer, you should accept that as a fact of life. Unlike the firms in many other industries, American bike companies have given up the low ground populated by generic ten-speeds or mountain bikes and have dominated the high-end categories, including mountain bikes, with and without suspension systems, and bikes made of nontraditional frame materials such as titanium, aluminum, carbon fiber, and a few others I'll mention later. As an American consumer shopping for a bike, you will be pleased to know that the majority of new ideas and innovative products are coming from tinkerers and companies in the States. In fact, mountain bikes designed and/or manufactured by Specialized, Trek, Cannondale, Mongoose, Marin, Fisher, and others have become the rage in Japan, Germany, England, and even Italy, which has seen its preeminence in bicycle innovation erode severely in the last 20 years.

So you can shop with some assurance that the multitude of bikes on display are likely American-designed and -inspired, if not American-made. You will quickly come to realize, however, that differentiation among and between bikes is most noticeable at the higher end. Many bikes around $300 can be essentially the same, with different logos, manufactured at the worthy Giant factory in Taiwan, the China Bicycle Company in China, or other places in the Far East. Bike shop personnel will have a difficult time differentiating at the lower price points, but that is their problem. You certainly can—and many millions do—buy a bike for $300 or less and can expect a responsive, reliable bike that will have a long life. You will pay for incremental improvements in weight, responsiveness, and performance, but I've never met a cyclist who said such a trade-off was not worth the money.

A QUESTION OF NEED

But first, do you need a new bike? Few American homes do not have a bike of some kind on the premises. I know; I've seen a lot of them. Many are still roadworthy. My brother has an original Raleigh team bike he purchased in Bangkok thirty years ago and reminds me that's all the bike he'll ever need, a sentiment I appreciate though I remind him it's bad for my image and my business. Anyway, my advice is not to run out and buy a new bike. If the bike you have is comfortable, weighs not much more than 30 pounds, has aluminum rather than steel rims (wheels), has low enough gearing, and can keep you in the saddle without discomfort, you're probably all right. If you are in doubt, you might want to visit your local bike shop. If you've had your bike more than 3 or 4 years, you might want to consider a trade-in, which most shops are open to. Or an upgrade, particularly of your gearing, which has changed significantly in the last few years now that the foolproof index shifting has become the norm. However, upgrades can be expensive, and in the long run it might be better for you to bite the bullet and get that new bike.

If you purchased your present bike at a department store and can afford to invest in a new one, I encourage you to do so. Frankly, though I have many good friends at Huffy, Roadmaster, and Murray, I would not buy these bikes for a serious fitness program. I don't want to be a snob about this. When I got to China, I was amazed, not only at the number of bikes but at the amount of produce, farm animals, and furniture the Chinese can transport on single-speed bikes. And I get little comfort in knowing Shimano, the Japanese component giant, plans to make every Chinese bike more than one-speed. I'm old enough to look back nostalgically on my Raleigh three-speed. For the Chinese, the bicycle, not the automobile, is what moves a population of one billion and is therefore an indispensable part of the transportation mix. Sadly, this is not so in America, where health and fitness are not sufficiently part of our web of life. So we must join health clubs and the like. I should note, without any apologies, that when I ask Chinese cyclists whether they'd rather have their one-speed Pigeon or a multispeed lightweight bike, they always choose the latter. So we should enjoy and profit from our technology. I want your cycling program to be a "walk in the park." Aficionados who joke about the bike feeling or being a part of them or the bike "disappearing beneath them" are not just engaging in hyperbole. That is precisely the feeling one gets on a bike that is lightweight, comfortable, and properly fitted.

One more thought before you decide to sell, toss, or upgrade your existing bike. I encourage you to think long and hard about the kind of cycling you will be doing, an exercise that will be easier after you finish this book. My experience is that most people who enter a bike shop with purchase in mind know little about the product and how they intend to use it. It's a sunny day in May, and you want to feel the wind in your hair. Slow down. More bikes have gone into early retirement because consumers didn't think about use.

If I've been asked this question once, I've been asked it a thousand times: "What bike should I buy?" If I know the questioner well, know his or her cycling habits and goals, and have some idea of the many available styles, I might say, "Well, you might have a look at the Specialized Stumpjumper or the Cannondale Delta V or the Trek 5500, bikes I know well and have used for years." And even then I would be reluctant to give quick or unsolicited advice without knowing more about the intended use of the bike. Typical call: "Hi. Is this the editor of *Mountain Bike*? Well, I'm Joe Savage, from Shelcota, Pennsylvania, and I'm going on this trip and was wondering if you'd suggest a bike."

WHICH BIKE?

I tell my secretary to hold my calls and ask the usual questions. "Are you an experienced cyclist? What was the last bike you owned? Weight, height? How many miles a day will you cycle on your trip? Will it be on-road or off-road? Hilly? Flat? With others? What kind of cycling will you do after your trip? How much money do you have to spend?" And on and on and on.

I participate in a lot of MS rides and have been responsible for raising a fair bit of money for this worthy cause. Some years ago my son, Declan, wanted to join me and I was delighted though concerned. He insisted on using his mountain bike. "Declan," I said, "you'll find the mountain bike comfortable for the first few miles, then you might have trouble keeping up," the rolling resistance being increased by the heavy knobby tires. No, he wouldn't listen and sure enough thirty miles into the ride he climbed aboard the sag wagon. My son is the rule rather than the exception. I am convinced millions of Americans are riding badly fitted bikes or bikes not suited to the riding purpose of both. These are the reasons so many bikes are parked in garages.

I'm intentionally making a fuss about this because I want every reader of this book to embrace cycling as a lifesport. To make that a reality, you must be sitting on the right bike, which might mean making some compromises. Let me explain.

In 1995 approximately 11 million bikes will be sold in the United States, about the same number as cars. Of that number, more than 60 percent will be mountain bikes, the rest hybrid or cross bikes, touring and fitness bikes, road-racing bikes, and a variety of bikes for children, including motocross. The adult consumer who walks into a specialty shop is faced with three categories of bikes: *mountain, road,* and *cross* or *hybrid,* actually a compromise version of the first two.

Some readers will remember that, as recently as 10 years ago, mountain bikes were unheard of in most sections of the country, parts of California and Colorado being the exceptions. American adult consumers had limited choices. You'd buy either a *racing bike,* literally modeled on what participants in the Tour de France used, high gearing and all; a *generic ten-speed,* based on the racing model and stamped out in factories in Japan and Taiwan; or a so-called *touring bike,* which looked like a racing bike but had lower gears and a longer wheel base (axle to axle measurement) for comfort. That was it. The generic ten-speeds were a joke. They were badly designed, machined, and assembled. No wonder when mountain bikes came on the scene, the generic ten-speed category disappeared overnight. Americans voted with their feet and wallets and for good reason. The ten-speeds were unreliable and had hard saddles, skinny tires, and crazy gearing with levers on the down tube only the long-armed could reach. On the other hand, the mountain bike had a more comfortable saddle, wider tires to cushion the ride, and gear shifts and brake levers on the handlebars within reach. No wonder the change. It didn't matter that fewer than 18 percent of all mountain bike purchasers ever rode their bike off-road, let alone in the mountains. This was a category that would stick and redefine the American and world bike markets.

If the mountain bike was an answer to the "underdesign" of the generic ten-speed, the hybrid or cross-bike is an answer to the overdesigned mountain bike. For example, you'll often find thicker, beefier frames on mountain bikes than your riding would require. The fat, knobby tires, though largely puncture-proof, slow you down. And overall the bike isn't very aerodynamic, increasing wind resistance, a not insignificant factor if you're interested in on-road cycling at speed.

The hybrid or cross-bike is a compromise. Manufacturers have borrowed from the traditional road bike using narrower tires than found on mountain bikes. Often a hybrid will have a version of the down-turned or drop bar. And the saddle is not quite as wide. This compromise bike allows you to ride on the road without a rolling resistance penalty but also permits you to ride trails and backroads, customary terrains of the mountain bike. Though this design is still evolving, the category accounts for about 20 percent of the adult bikes sold through specialty shops and is increasing every year, so clearly the hybrid has found a market. Univega, Schwinn, and Bianchi have led the way in manufacturing these new bikes.

So what bike should you buy? Mary Ann Duckert of Waukesha, Wisconsin, a grandmother, tells me she owns a road bike (drop handlebars), a hybrid (flat handlebars), a mountain bike, and a recumbent—the kind of bike you sit down in to pedal. This "bike Grandma" cycles about 4,000 miles a year, starting with short rides, then hills and into the wind. She finds trail riding good for building endurance, adding, "Sometimes a 10-mile ride is better than a 50 for training, if it's done on the trail."

Findley Gillespie of Woodinville, Washington, owns a road and a mountain bike, and hates hybrids. He says, "They aren't good road bikes or good mountain bikes. Just pieces of junk."

For others it's a seasonal decision. Jan Wagner of Hastings, Michigan, rides his mountain bike 5 days a week from November to March. From April to October, he rides his road bike 6 days a week.

Cyclists frequently tell me they use their mountain bikes for family and social riding and their road bikes for fitness training and performance riding. Others, like John Boone, of Machias, Maine, rides his mountain bike more for general transportation and group rides in the summer.

In other words, you'll find as many preferences as you will find cyclists. Some are passionately devoted to the road bike and others to the mountain or hybrid bike. My guess is that, as you become committed to cycling, you'll probably discover you'll want a road bike and mountain bike or hybrid because cycling is a year-round activity and different bikes better suit the weather, road conditions, and your mood.

I'm writing this during the Blizzard of '93. I live on a small farm and have cut mountain bike trails through and around the property. Most of the fall and winter I'm on my Barricuda or Raleigh mountain bikes. Certainly I'm getting training but that's not the primary reason I ride mountain bikes. I do so to be part of and one with the environment. I like to get close to the native grasses that grow here, to see deer and the occasional fox, to watch our "pet" kestrel, to be surprised by bear scat. Yes, I go on mountain bike rides in Colorado, California, and other places, but these rides close to my home are most precious and in some way sacred to me. The poet Robert Bly has said man has a responsibility to know the plants, trees, and animals around him by name as well as by intuition. The mountain bike allows me to do that, though I fully recognize there are those who blow through the landscape without smelling the roses and are still riding responsibly.

I love my mountain bikes and would not like to choose between them and a road bike. Though I ride a mountain bike throughout the year, I consider it an adjunct to my conditioning program. For example, right now I'm preparing for a 1,000-mile ride across the South of France, with a friend. The mountain bike is very much a part of my

19

off-season training program. Within a month or so, I'll be back on my road bike, a Trek 5500, to prepare for my long tour. Of course, I could use a mountain bike on my French tour; people do. I saw plenty of mountain bikes on my Land's End to John o' Groat's trip. On querying, I usually discovered that these cyclists were doing 30–40 miles a day, moving along at their own good pace. Good luck to them; that's their preference. Still, for a fast, efficient workout on tour, the road bike is your best choice.

I know. It sounds as if I'm pushing you toward becoming a two-bike household before you have the first one paid off. That's not my intention. I simply want you to know the options.

Under ideal circumstances, you'd be a more complete cyclist with prospects for year-round training if you had both a road and a mountain bike. If, like most, you have to choose, use the following as a guideline: If you are buying and riding a bike primarily for fitness, health, weight control, and the like, and you are or expect to become a reasonably competent cyclist with little concern about traffic, I recommend you buy a road bike. This choice would be particularly sound if you have quick and easy access to good roads and you plan to cap off your season with a long tour or century ride (100 miles), usually considered a mark of accomplishment for the recreational cyclist.

If you are more comfortable on a bike with flat (vs. downturned) handlebars and are willing to sacrifice a little speed and responsiveness for potential comfort, you might want a hybrid or cross-bike. This choice would make even more sense if you intended to do some of your cycling off-road on trails, dirt paths, or single tracks. It won't give you the performance of a road bike but would be adequate for your training schedule.

The mountain bike speaks for itself. Some cyclists I know have never been on any other kind of bike. The arguments offered for considering a road or hybrid would likely be scoffed at by some of my colleagues who would argue a mountain bike is equally comfortable in any terrain. I hear that remark most often by cyclists who live in California, Colorado, or other places within spitting distance of a great single track. But this is not a contest; not an either/or situation. If you intend to ride primarily off-road on logging trails and single track, the mountain bike is definitely for you. Keep in mind that 60 percent of the bikes sold in the United States are mountain bikes, so the cycling population has already voted.

Let me summarize some pluses and minuses.

Mountain: All-around, versatile; they do it all (almost): trail riding, off-road racing, commuting, touring. *Plus:* Comfortable upright riding position; shock-absorbing and flat resistant tires; easy-to-reach controls; strong frame, fork and wheels; low gears; low maintenance. *Minus:* Upright position and wide tires make bike slower and harder to pedal long distances; usually heavier than road bikes; fewer hand positions than with drop bars.

Hybrid: Features upright riding position and convenient controls of mountain bikes; narrower tires better suited for pavement. Note: There were 149 hybrid models offered in 1992, 126 in 1994. *Plus:* Good commuting bike; good on-road and off; comfortable; flat resistant tires, good braking; can carry loads. *Minus:* Upright position not aerodynamic; heavier than a road bike; fewer hand positions; less control off-road than on a mountain bike; slower on pavement than a road bike.

Road: Often called road-racing bike though something of a misnomer. Drop handlebars allow different hand positions for comfort. Aerodynamic posture. *Plus:* Lightweight; most efficient riding position for power; quick handle; best for fast recreational riding. *Minus:* Tires more susceptible to puncture; may need to experiment with seats to get comfortable; takes time to adapt to riding position.

By now you should have a fairly good idea of what bike or bikes best suit your needs. No need to rush your purchase; the average consumer visits at least four bike shops before he or she makes a decision. Women often are forced to go farther afield because selections for them are still not what they should be, a matter I will take up shortly.

These days, even in the smallest bike shops you'll have a choice of major brands. You might find Trek, Giant, Univega, and Raleigh in one store; Cannondale, Schwinn, Diamondback, and GT in another. The logic varies. Gone are the days when the old Schwinn company could insist their dealers primarily carry Schwinns. Retailers have gotten a lot more independent and the brands they carry often depend on what moves in the neighborhood and what a competitive shop is carrying. Don't be surprised to find bikes ranging from $250 to $2,500. This wide range has less to do with marketing hype and more to do with the tremendous variety of bikes offered. It's not uncommon for our annual Buyer's Guide in *Bicycling* and *Mountain Bike* to publish information on more than a thousand models offered by ninety companies. There are also more than seventy custom builders who make fine custom-built bikes. Here's some advice for the novice bike buyer:

1. Do most of your shopping before you enter the store.
2. Know what local stores carry which brands.
3. Have a firm price range in mind.
4. Buy nothing until you road-test the product under real life conditions. Enlightened stores encourage this. If your shop does not, make for the door.
5. Don't be rushed into any purchase. You'll have plenty of time to regret it.
6. Beware of buying too much bike. As you read this book, suspension systems are the rage for mountain bikes and even showing up on road bikes. Before you buy a suspension bike, take a dual-suspension bike on a good climb. Repeat.

If you still are confused about the broad array of brands on the showroom floor, listen to cycling enthusiasts about their brand choices. According to *Bicycling*'s 1994 Subscriber Study, the top 10 brands of bicycles owned in order are: Trek, Schwinn, Specialized, Cannondale, Raleigh, Giant, Nishiki, Bianchi, Diamondback, and Fuji. GT was right behind Fuji.

According to the same study, the top road/sport bikes are perceived to be: Trek, Cannondale, Specialized, Bianchi, Schwinn, Eddy Merckx, Kestrel, Merlin, Serotta, and Klein.

The top mountain bikes are: Trek, Cannondale, Specialized, Diamondback, GT, Giant, Bridgestone, Klein, Marin, Schwinn, and Fisher.

The top hybrid/cross-bikes are: Trek, Schwinn, Specialized, Giant, Cannondale, Raleigh, Bianchi, Diamondback, Nishiki, GT, Univega, and Fuji.

I haven't mentioned tandems but here are the top five: Cannondale, Burley, Santana, Trek, and Schwinn.

When asked what brands they would consider for their next purchase, readers responded: Trek, Cannondale, Specialized, Giant, Schwinn, Bridgestone, Diamondback, Bianchi, Raleigh, and Merlin.

What does this mean? Simply, 2 million readers who are knowledgeable about the sport and who have been influenced by *Bicycling* magazine, friends, and advertisements (in that order) have made brand choices and recommendations that are remarkably consistent. Keep in mind that these readers represent the enthusiast end of the market and are 70 percent male. In surveys I have conducted of a cross section of the American population, Schwinn, Huffy, and Murray top the list of brands owned. Schwinn's position can be explained by its 100-year dominance in the American market, and Huffy and Murray tend to serve the large lower-end market of Infrequent riders, who spend on the average about $140 for a new bike.

Since I'm recommending you make your purchase from a specialty shop, the first set of brand-name suggestions and recommendations are the best guidelines, with a few caveats.

Schwinn, traditionally a road bike company, has come back strong, after going through Chapter 11, in the mountain bike field. The company moved its offices to Colorado to be close to the sport. So Schwinn's numbers don't reflect the full strength and diversity of its line.

GT is probably understated, having started as a BMX company, but it has moved aggressively into the mountain bike market. Furthermore, it just launched a road/sport bike line with an eye to the 1996 Olympics.

Cannondale, one of the most innovative bike companies in the world, is making an even stronger commitment to the mountain bike field, underscored by a joint venture with Magic Motorcycles.

You won't go wrong buying any of the brands I suggest, but please keep an eye out for the "smaller" brands such as Marin, Mongoose, Univega Fisher (now an independent company within the Trek organization), Univega, and others that enter the market on a regular basis.

COMPONENT PARTS

So you have your needs in order, brands in head, cash in hand, and you trip over an odd assortment of steel, titanium, aluminum, carbon fiber, and composite bikes fresh from the space program. What's a body to do?

For one thing, don't go kicking the tires. You might get sucked in by an erstwhile clerk to lifting the bikes and "oohing" and "aahing" about their incredible lightness of being. I don't know why but that seems to be everyone's first inclination from England to Iran to China. The light in the eyes is all the same.

Let's get back to basics. Steel has been around a long time, and pound for pound it's our most durable, resilient, reliable metal. Armies have moved by bike, as have livestock and entire communities. It will rarely fail you. Sure it rusts if you leave it out in monsoon rains and can become fatigued after a crash or long wear.

Steel bikes have been around for a hundred years and will likely be around for another hundred. Naturally, there is a certain nostalgia for this metal. I recall talking to Antonio Columbo of Columbus tubing, the venerable Italian tube manufacturing company that has been supplying frame materials to the best racers for generations. This was about the time carbon fiber had become popular. Columbo was adamant about the superior properties of steel and the continuing advances made in the alloying of the metal. To be sure, fewer and fewer custom makers are producing bikes out of straight, traditional tubes, primarily for performance and not marketing reasons.

But talk to anyone producing nonferrous bikes and you'll get a different story. Engineers who design Kestrel frames believe that the bike industry will go the way of golf, skiing, and tennis; composite materials will push the older metals out of the industry. And I've heard the same arguments applied many times to titanium and aluminum bikes.

Over the years, I've seen, as manufacturers rush to market or to gain a competitive edge, a fair number of shoddy aluminum, titanium, and carbon-fiber bikes. Until Cannondale mastered the beefy, thick-tubed aluminum frame, I found most aluminum bikes lacked stiffness. Likewise at *Bicycling* we discovered our share of bonded bikes that became unglued. And titanium parts that have cracked.

However, technical advances, a competitive marketplace, and an increasingly sophisticated consumer guarantee that the bikes you see on a showroom floor are safe, ridable, and guaranteed.

In our *Bicycling* test lab we have an assortment of equipment to measure the variances formed and stresses applied when you ride, particularly when you cycle hard. Watch the cyclist in front of you when he or she is climbing a hill, out of the saddle, rocking back and forth, putting tremendous pressure (load) on the pedals and bottom bracket. We can measure that.

We can measure how much shock absorption or dampening effect the various suspension systems have and how that affects cycling over various surfaces. And we frequently work with the engineers at the General Motors wind tunnel to find ways to make the bicycle and the rider more aerodynamic because, in the long run, wind resistance is your biggest obstacle to going faster.

A lot of our analysis is at the margins. For example, you'll go faster if you shave your legs, wear skin tight clothing, and use aero bars. I'm talking fractions of a second, measures that make a great difference to the racers and, as you get more serious about a training program, will make a difference to you.

There are computer printouts of the specifications and riding qualities of most bikes in America. Ultimately, however, the choice is very personal and often comes down to how you feel on a bike. And in part this will depend on your weight, riding style, fitness, and performance goals.

If you enter a bike shop and say: "I have three hundred dollars and want to buy a basic bike that will enable me to commute, ride around the neighborhood, and build a fitness program around," the clerk might say, "Here's the ideal bike for you, a Univega Expresso, a hybrid bike, made of steel, weighing thirty pounds."

Remember that 67 percent of the mountain bikes sold have steel frames, a percentage not likely to change in this century. The most affordable bikes on the market, all made of steel, in the various categories are: Mountain bike—$170; mountain bike with front suspension—$309; mountain bike with front and rear suspension—$649; road/sport bike—$280; and hybrid—$190. The price range of bikes on the market today is vast, however—from $170 to $8,000. You pay for light weight, for performance, and for hand-crafted, better-machined products. You have to decide how much bike is necessary to provide a comfortable ride and meet your fitness and performance goals.

As I write this, I'm already seeing prototypes of bikes that will be on the market long after you read this. Bikes marketed in the mid-nineties will be lighter, with more consumer extras such as bar-end shifters and advanced shifting technology, than bikes available today.

Whatever name you find on the top tube or downtube of a bike, signifying the manufacturer, one name will show up on many bikes, and that is Shimano, a components manufacturer. By my count, Shimano gearing is presently on 90 percent of all mountain bikes, with and without suspension, 45 percent of all road/sport bikes, and 87 percent of all hybrids, giving it a dominant—even monolithic—presence in the American market. You'll see "names" such as STX, LX, XT, and XTR, denoting Shimano component groups in different ranges. By the time you read this, Shimano's influence will have lessened, but it will still be formidable.

Generally speaking, higher prices mean better bearings, more aluminum alloy (vs. stamped steel and plastic), lighter weight, more powerful brakes, and stronger cold-forged parts. I have done more discrete analysis showing how much money you spend for each gram of weight improvement. With few (if any) exceptions, if you spend more for a lightweight, responsive bike, you will get more enjoyment out of cycling and more fitness from your bike. Road-test them. You'll certainly be able to tell the difference between a $300 Tourney-equipped Schwinn and a $600 STX-equipped Trek. The shifting on the latter will be quicker, crisper, and much more responsive, and these qualities are not insignificant if you plan to ride 4–5 times a week. Indeed, you want a bike that is light and responsive so you can spend the time worrying about your body, not your bike. I mean, after this chapter, I want to say little about the bike itself. So do me a favor and buy the best bike you can afford so I'll look good and so will you.

Let me summarize. If you intend to tool around town, you can buy any bike from the lower end of the spectrum and get some satisfaction. But for a bike that is to become a centerpiece of your fitness and health program, I'd recommend you start your search at $400. By and large, when you get much over $1,000, subtlety takes over and it's hard to put a price tag on the esoteric. Keep in mind that since many of the components come from the same source, price differences in similarly equipped models will often reflect in the quality of the frame and fork.

I'm not going to say much about single or dual suspension mountain bikes. Every year more mountain bikes and now some road bikes are offered with suspension systems, with Rock Shocks leading the market. There's a lot of hype in this category and consumers continue to buy too much technology for their needs. You don't need a suspended bike for riding on roads, bike paths, and fairly even trails. You might want to consider one if you intend to race mountain bikes, especially downhill, intend to do most of your riding off-road, or have a regular diet of bumpy, washboard terrain. Or if you have a bad back.

And you do pay a weight penalty. Fully suspended mountain bikes still weigh up to four pounds more than their unsuspended cousin, a weight differential that is punishingly significant, especially when climbing hills. For a fitness program, you want the lightest bike you can afford. I advise you not to load it down with unnecessary technology. Fortunately for the consumer, suspension technology gets lighter and more affordable by the year and is beginning to show up on road bikes.

Keep in mind that you are buying a consumer product, not something precious, and be ready to shop around. The most popular months for buying bikes are May, June, and December. Beat the spring rush and make your purchase in January or February when there's a lot of inventory to be cleared out. Some shops will offer trade-ins, but as with a car, you'll get a better price for the old model if you sell it yourself.

You should now be ready to buy a bike, but before you straddle that machine, we'll talk about fit, a subject worthy of the next chapter. As I've said before, in my opinion, the primary reason people do not ride their bike is the bikes don't fit.

Remember the cyclist quoted earlier who said it should be a felony for a shop to sell a customer an ill-fitting bike? Well, I'm in the crime prevention business.

FIT

You don't have to be an expert to spot a novice cyclist or one who just pulled a bike out of the box. Too often the saddle is low, legs sticking out akimbo, like disconnected wings. The cyclist is probably pushing a gearing that is too high because he heard somewhere that you have to pedal slow and hard to get maximum benefit from the sport.

I don't exaggerate. Look carefully at the cyclists you see in the next few days. Notice the children riding bikes that are too large for them, purchased or handed down with the false notion that the young body will grow into the bike as into old shoes.

Look at women on bikes with a too long top tube, a frequent occurrence because manufacturers still do not provide an acceptable range of products for women. Note the cyclists who push their bikes up even a moderate grade, a practice not so much dictated by lack of fitness, though that can play a part, but by the high gearing that manufacturers still put on products. I was in good shape before my ride across Britain but I still had to put on three lower gears before the ride. Manufacturers are still too influenced by the racing scene.

And finally, note the unused bikes in garages and basements around the neighborhood, a tribute to the bike industry that has spent too much time worrying about volume and not enough on sizing bikes for the physiologies of a real population.

Quite true, you can jump on any old bike and cycle to the store or friends' homes. No damage done. Kids do this all the time with few ill effects. But for the adult who plans to make the bike the centerpiece of a fitness program, approximate fit is not good enough. If you are to make maximum use of your bike, the bike should fit you like a glove. In effect, the bike becomes an extension of you, a part of your physiology. You and the bicycle join in a special biomechanics, unique to you. Appropriate attention to fit now will pay dividends the rest of your cycling life.

Another good reason for buying a bike at a specialty shop is that here and here alone will you find skilled salesmen and cyclists who will pay proper attention to fit. Few shops will haggle about making changes in parts and components, such as saddle, seat post, and stem, if the changes make you more comfortable on a bike.

As it's easy to tell a cyclist on an ill-fitting bike, it's just as easy to spot a cyclist who is properly fitted. Whether looking at Lance Armstrong, American World Champion, or Juli Furtado, World Champion Mountain Biker, you'll note that they are one with the bike, sitting comfortably and relaxed in the saddle, set to accelerate when provoked. The aim is a relaxed riding position, whether you're on a mountain, sport bike, or hybrid. Here are some tips on getting the proper fit.

MOUNTAIN BIKE

1. Frame. Let's assume you are indeed riding the trails, the single track as they are called, and you choose to stop and dismount rather than jump over a log. For that reason and many others, you'll want significant clearance between your crotch and the top tube, perhaps up to a couple of inches. Keep in mind that the ideal size of a mountain bike might be 2–3 inches smaller than your road bike size. Because a lot of bike manufacturers list frame sizes in metric, I've included a conversion table in the Appendixes. When I refer to frame size, I'm referring to the measurement from the center of the crank axle to the center of the top tube. Some manufacturers specify frame sizes in other ways such as from the crank axle to the top of the top tube or to the top of an extended seat lug. Further complicating matters is that some mountain bikes have curved top tubes and shorter-

than-average seat tubes. So a mountain bike with a 16-inch seat tube might be perfect for someone who rides a 23-inch road bike. *Please don't be confused by any of these measurements.* Just make sure you and the salesperson are talking about the same thing. Know that a smaller mountain bike frame is an advantage because it's stiffer, lighter, and more manageable. I ride a 59 cm road frame (23.2 inches, crank axle to bottom bracket) but am quite comfortable on mountain bikes of 54 cm (20.3 inches) and smaller. The smaller frame size allows me to get over the bike more, to feel in control, and to change my center of gravity often, a vital skill in this sport.

2. <u>Saddle Height</u>. Seat posts are sufficiently long that you can raise them 5–6 inches before the maximum extension line shows. When pedaling, your knee should be slightly bent at the bottom of the stroke. Let this position come naturally. A lot of cyclists tend to drop a heel at the bottom of the stroke, extending the leg too far. I frequently see cyclists with so much extension that they rock from side to side in the saddle.

One of the first tricks I learned the hard way about mountain biking was to lower the saddle for rough terrain, taking a little pressure off the crotch. I recall some early rides in the mountains around Crested Butte, Colorado, filming a segment for *Good Morning America.* I learned quick from the experts that I should drop my saddle even lower for steep descents, though at times, I still had to literally sit on the rear wheel to keep my weight lower and far enough back. But these are skills you will learn on the bike. Make sure the seat post has enough extension that your cycling needs will be met. Please don't be reluctant to ask for the seat post to be removed from the seat tube for your inspection.

3. <u>Top Tube and Stem Length</u>. If your photograph were taken on a mountain bike, the result you'd want to see is a straight back with arms comfortably bent. Mountain bikes have extralong seat posts, for reasons stated above, so it's often the top tube length rather than seat tube length that is the determining factor whether to buy a smaller or larger frame size. To be sure, once you've purchased a bike, you'll experiment on the "road" with the components of fit—that is to be expected. However, the bicycle should be fitted to you before you leave the shop. Don't accept the frequently heard remark, especially if you're a woman, that "your body will get used to it." That has some truth as far as the saddle is concerned, but even here an initial test ride will be revealing.

4. Handlebar Width and Sweep. From end to end, 21–24 inches between bars is common. If you want to be more aerodynamic, you'll want a narrower bar. If you want more slow-speed control, a wider bar is in order. Conventional advice suggests you can trim bars with a hacksaw to your physiological comfort. My advice is to leave a shop with the handlebar of your choice.

Handlebars come with varying degrees of rearward sweep, up to 12 degrees as a rule though I've seen sweep as much as 22 degrees. Sit on the bike, ride it, and determine your most comfortable hand and wrist position. A greater sweep probably changes your reach to the grips and controls and could necessitate a different stem length.

5. Stem Height and Rise. For maximum control and comfort, the stem should position the bar an inch or so below the saddle. This puts the weight on the front wheel, moving your center of gravity forward so it's easier to climb and less likely to pull up.

6. Fore/Aft Saddle Position. Since the saddle is the point where most body meets the bike, this is a subject I will—and you will—keep coming back to. Depending on the terrain, your fitness level, and your particular ride objectives, you will be fiddling with your saddle from time to time. But before you leave the shop, the fore/aft position should be adjusted. Some shops eyeball it; some use a fit kit or similar commercial measures; some use a plumb line. I'll use the latter for illustration. Sit comfortably on the saddle with crank arms horizontal. A plumb line dropped from just below the knee should intersect the pedal axis. If it doesn't, slide the saddle to achieve this. Keep in mind the preceding is a rule of thumb. Gonzo mountain bike riders who specialize in hill climbs push their saddles farther forward so they can sit on the plush part rather than the skinny neck. Such riders would also use a longer stem to keep the body from being cramped. But that's a specialty need.

7. <u>Crank Arm Length</u>. As a rule, crank arm length varies with frame size. For greater leverage on steep climbs, mountain bike cranks are usually 5 mm longer than road bike cranks. But unless you plan to do a lot of off-road hill climbing, I wouldn't worry too much about the crank length.

ROAD/SPORT BIKE

Not surprisingly, many of the "fit" features for the road bike are similar to the mountain bike. However, there are enough differences to warrant separate treatment.

1. <u>Frame</u>. As novices tend to ride larger frame sizes than their bodies warrant, enthusiasts prefer smaller frames because they are lighter, stiffer, and more responsive. Here's the frame sizing rule of thumb. Measure your inseam, crotch to floor, with bare feet 6 inches apart, and multiply by 0.65. That's it—your ideal road size frame, measured along the seat tube from the center of the crank axle to the center of the top tube. A double check should show about 4 inches of exposed seat post when your saddle height is correct.

You can do this measurement before you go shopping for a bike and then be reasonably certain of your frame size before you enter the door. The more of these simple but sometimes arcane measurements you master before hearing "Can I help you?", the better.

2. <u>Saddle Height</u>. The distance from the center of the bottom bracket to the top of the saddle should be 0.885 of inseam length, as measured in the previous example. As with the mountain bike, knees should be bent slightly at the bottom of the pedal stroke, the foot and pedal horizontal to the ground. Though a friend or a video camera will have to note, your hips should not rock when viewed from behind, a fairly common event as most new cyclists tend to have their saddles too high to get, one gathers, maximum benefit from the exercise.

If you have large feet for your size, you might want to raise the saddle slightly, say 2 mm. A good rule of thumb is to make saddle height changes in increments of 1 mm. Yes, a slight adjustment makes that much difference in your biomechanics.

3. Top Tube and Stem Length. My rule of thumb is this: I know when the top tube and stem length are correct when the front hub is obscured by the handlebar when I'm seated with hands on the brake hoods. Like other rules of thumb, consider this a starting point. The result you want is a comfortable riding position with a straight back and arms slightly bent. With experience, some road cyclists opt for a more extended, aerodynamic position by using a stem 1 or even 2 cm longer than the above formula suggests. Keep in mind that a shorter stem will give you more control and confidence in the beginning. You might never need to change.

4. Handlebar Width. Rule of thumb: Bar width should equal shoulder width. (Bars are available in 38-, 40-, and 42-cm widths.) Another rule of thumb: Go with the slightly wider bars to open your chest for breathing. The bottom, flat portion of the downturned handlebar should be level or pointed slightly down toward the rear hub. If you like a bike but don't feel comfortable with the handlebars, please ask for a change.

5. Stem Height. For most types of riding, the stem should be slightly below the top of the saddle, perhaps up to an inch. Racers might lower the stem as much as 2 inches below the saddle for improved aerodynamics, but such a position is not recommended for the fitness rider who wants to be comfortable but still get an exhilarating workout. You'll know when the time comes to lower the stem. That's serious business in more ways than one.

6. Fore/Aft Saddle Position. Same rule of thumb as for mountain bikes: The acronym KOPS (knee over pedal spindle) will help. This is considered the neutral position and quite comfortable for 95 percent of all recreational cyclists. As you progress, you might want to move the saddle aft slightly to get more leverage, especially in the hills. But I recommend you leave the store with the saddle in the neutral position.

7. Crank Arm Length. Rule of thumb: If your inseam is less than 29 inches, use a 165 mm crank arm; 29–32 inches, 170 mm; 32–34 inches, 172.5; and more than 24 inches, 175 mm. Crank arm length is measured from the center of the fixing bolt to the center of the pedal mounting hole. I've found this rule of thumb to hold up over time. My inseam measurement is 32 inches and I'm most comfortable on a 172.5 mm crank. I have gone up to 175 mm but never felt at home. I found I got better leverage but at the expense of pedaling speed, revolutions per minute (rpm), where much of the fitness and performance lies.

HYBRIDS

Hybrids (or cross or fitness bikes) usually have flat handlebars but are similar to road bikes in many respects. Therefore, you can apply many of the criteria offered above. If you do intend to ride the hybrid predominantly off-road, you might want to choose a smaller frame size. Keep in mind that some hybrids have higher bottom brackets (for clearance) than road bikes, so the standover height will be less for the same size frame. Two inches of clearance between crotch and frame are desirable.

Women should be particularly careful, no matter what bike they buy. As I've mentioned a number of times, the bike industry still does not provide a sufficient range of off-the-shelf products for women. Fortunately, more and more specialty shops are catering to women. If you're a woman shopping for a bike, you might want to confer with a female cyclist about her experiences.

A man and a woman of equal height won't necessarily fit on the same frame because women tend to have longer legs and shorter torsos. Not surprisingly, women find men's frames too long for their reach. Sometimes a shorter stem is the answer. Similarly, since women's shoulders are usually not as wide as men's, handlebars on off-the-shelf buys are often too wide, a situation that can be easily remedied by replacing them with narrower handlebars.

Given the fact that women's hands are usually smaller than men's, women should make sure their hands can reach the brakes or shift levers. For a mountain bike, sometimes a tapered bar is in order.

I've asked the American consumer what are the most important determinants when purchasing a bike, and here's the response: Reputation of manufacturer, reputation of dealer, dealer recommendation, made in America, made outside America, component selection, low weight, color/graphics, fit, comfort, frame design and materials, guarantee. These answers are from a random cross section of the American population, measuring according to *Bicycling* magazine, the opinions of four clusters of cyclists who exhibit different levels of enthusiasm for the sport: Enthusiast, Near Enthusiast, Casual Cyclist, and Infrequent Cyclist. I discovered that the more committed one becomes to cycling, the more important fit and comfort are. Even the Infrequent Cyclist who rides on the average 40 miles during the warm months recognizes that fit and comfort are important to successful cycling.

Consumers in search of a new bicycle tend to shop around, visiting an average of four bikes shops. One reason for this is difficulty finding a bike that fits. I asked consumers, "Did you have trouble finding a bicycle with the right fit or frame size?" Most had difficulty finding a bike that fit, indicating particularly for the latter group of 25 million who shop at the mass merchants, that they would be better off shopping at a specialty store.

Bike fit, especially saddle height, might be the most controversial area in cycling, perhaps fueled by a scene in the classic cycling film, *A Sunday in Hell,* in which Belgium great Eddy Merckx is shown frequently adjusting his saddle. I've seen cyclists do the same thing as Sunday riders, adjusting saddle height for changes in the wind and atmosphere pressure. After a point, all this gets silly. There are countless other ways to fit your body to the bike, all containing a degree of truth. The United States Cycling team has a method, so does Eddy Borysewicz, former U.S. Olympic coach, and so does the guy next door. The more enlightened bike shop might have the New England Cycling Academy Fit Kit or Serotta's Fit Cycle to scientifically match the rider to the bike. The Fit Kit system, developed by Bill Farrell and used by a thousand bike shops, was created by averaging scores of top riders' physical dimensions and their bike setups, producing a recommended range. I've used the Fit Kit and other systems and found they generally replicate what my experience and rule of thumb tell me. The Fit Kit is particularly helpful if you think a different crank arm or longer stem is in order.

Still, whether you use the rules of thumb presented here, which are quite reliable, the eyes of an Olympic coach, or a Fit Kit, all these systems are static and don't tell you what's happening when you are actually pedaling, bending your ankles, and shifting around on the saddle. Researchers have developed a motion analysis technique that videotapes the pedal stroke from three views. The tape is converted into a stick figure on a computer screen and the various angles can be measured. Generally, computer analysis, which is becoming much more available at sports medicine clinics, seems most useful for the elite racer and cyclists with severe biomechanical imbalances. But if you feel the need and have access to such a system, take advantage of it.

Later we will talk about using the very down-home video camera for improving your cycling techniques. Computer simulation, while interesting, is best left to the Olympic cyclist. We'll try to keep our bike riding simple.

We've been in the bike shop too long. You have the bike of your dream. You have so harangued the salesperson that he or she has changed stem, crank, and handlebars in the interest of your comfort. Finally, the bike fits you and your style of riding. The bike is responsive and light enough to be a passport to health and fitness.

Let's get on the road and trails.

C·H·A·P·T·E·R T·H·R·E·E

SKILLS

One truism I'm tired of hearing is, "You never forget how to ride a bike." Perhaps, but the statement masks how most people actually learn. On this matter, I'm no different from other parents. I taught my daughter to ride by gently pushing her down a grassy knoll, time and time again, until she gained confidence and decided to come to an elegant stop rather than fall. No damage done. She wore a helmet, gloves, and knee pads and remembers the event fondly. Since that time, we've cycled regularly. Now, as a teenager, she has her eyes on a car and I'm afraid my instructions must wait a few years. She'll come back.

Not long ago, I learned to scuba dive, or rather, relearned an activity I first tried when stationed with the Navy in the Pacific. I loved it. When I returned to the sport, I was struck with the education process, a week of classroom study, pool activity, and open water (ocean) diving. To be sure, scuba is a potentially dangerous activity, though in practice very safe. The training is necessary because you dive with air tanks and a regulator. In other words, you depend on a mechanical system to breathe. So training is vital.

With scuba (an acronym for self-contained underwater breathing apparatus), once you get the breathing and buoyancy control down pat, everything else is easy. For most that means diving in the deep blue water of the Caribbean.

With cycling, you're moving through another kind of space, over varying terrain, in the company of other cyclists or traffic, in a variety

39

of weather conditions. In diving, one has the current to contend with; in cycling it's the wind. In diving, the less energy you expend (or the less air you breathe), the more efficient you are. With cycling, the opposite is true. You *want* to expend energy. While cycling can be as relaxing as scuba diving, if you ride for health, fitness, and performance, you will raise your pulse.

My golfing friends talk often about the instruction they receive in order to shave a few strokes off a handicap. My skiing friends chat about the annual instruction they receive when returning to the slopes. And my tennis friends are always in and out of clinics. The backhand, you know.

But cycling, the largest and fastest-growing recreational activity in the country, has really no endemic instruction waiting for us when we purchase a bike. Ironically, the sport that has the most equipment, involves the most complex biomechanics, and can potentially put the participant at risk, has little or no formal instruction. That task is left to friends, magazines, and books. To be sure, instructional cycling camps are becoming increasingly popular in response to the call for personal coaching, but most are expensive, require travel, and last a week or longer. Although a camp such as Carpenter/Phinney, run by two fine instructors—ex-racers and colleagues—might be in your future, my position is that you can indeed be your own coach, trainer, therapist, and even "psychologist." Over the last decade or so I've met, interviewed, read about, or been exposed to the best coaches and trainers in the business. Similarly, I've been associated with the cream of professional and amateur cyclists who have readily offered their technical advice. Furthermore, I've had the pleasure of learning from many thousands of recreational cyclists who really do "live to cycle and cycle to live." I believe you can rise to the top of your fitness and form by listening to your body and taking charge of your training program. How you sit on, ride, use, handle, trust, push, and take care of your bike will say a lot about your own health.

Though you can question my math, given what I've written so far, I submit that cycling is one-tenth mechanical and nine-tenths physical relating to skills. Perhaps you've already seen two cyclists riding similar bikes but the difference is apparent. Comfort, riding ability, ease of

40

pedaling, and general cycling demeanor can vary like night and day. The determining factor is technique, something everyone can learn.

Whether watching champion Lance Armstrong on the road, or Juli Furtado on the single track, what they have in common is "bike ease," the ease with which they sit on, handle, and fall into their bikes. They are truly one with their bikes and it shows.

At this point, I'm assuming you have a bike, it fits you like a glove, and you know how to turn the pedals. You know that there is less resistance when you're in the smallest chainring, commonly used for climbing hills or riding into a head wind. You've already moved the chain through the cogs or sprockets and know that the smaller cogs are for descending and flatland riding and the larger cogs for climbing. Now all these gearing decisions are made easier because many new bikes have optical displays telling you what gear you are in.

Don't be reluctant to go to a quiet street or parking lot to play. The majority of casual cyclists use no more than a few gears on a multiple-speed bike. Consider the gears part of your physiology, like your legs or heart, because these muscles signal you when to shift into a higher or lower gear. These days, especially with mountain bikes, the gear shifters are push-button and numbered, making it very easy to know where you are. Foolproof gear shifting is here. So take the time to learn your bikes.

Don't laugh, but some cyclists even tape a gear chart on the stem so they know exactly what gear they are in. I include a table and formula in the Appendixes. This is a useful exercise, whether you put a chart on the stem or not. But by actually counting teeth on the cogs or chainrings and converting them to inches, you will know whether your bike is geared correctly—it is not unusual for a 21-speed bike to have 5–6 gears that are so close they are practically useless. In this vein, don't be bowled over by the 21-speed marketing hype you hear on the showroom floor. First of all, you don't need that many gears. Second, the bike probably doesn't have 21 discrete gears anyway. Third, the bike often is biased toward high gears, lacking the low gears that are essential for an all-around, all-terrain training program. The right gearing is an indispensable ally as you develop proper technique. Unfortunately, since you can't always tell until you ride the bike for a few weeks, have an understanding with the salesperson, in writing, that you can bring the bike back for a change in gearing as part of your free 30-day checkup. Usually the procedure consists of no more than changing a chainring or a cog or two. But exercise that right. With the advent of indexing and handlebar-mounted levers, it's easier than ever to shift often, as you should. The right, properly spaced gearing will allow you to do just that. Remember the best cyclists shift often, responding to every increase in elevation and wind resistance. Only the foolhardy pick high gears to show how tough they are. Cycling is a sport of elegance, subtly, and finesse. Proper use of the right gearing is part of that elegance.

Recall your first bike ride or your child's. Most of us tend to grip the bike as if it will run away, instead of sitting on it gently, holding the bars firmly, not fiercely. One secret to getting the most from your cycling is to ride softly, using your gears and brakes as if they are an extension of you, which is exactly what they are.

As more than one cyclist will tell you, cycling is not about being big, being strong, being a Big Man on Campus. In fact, what draws many men and women to cycling is that they don't have to be star athletes or even close. Though one's ability to metabolize oxygen and natural athletic ability can separate champions from the runner-ups, for the fitness cyclist skill makes all the difference. For this book I interviewed thousands of cyclists of all ages, backgrounds and abilities, and not surprisingly, 90 percent of them ride most of the time alone, though acknowledge they would ride more if they had someone to ride with. My point is that cycling, though a social activity, is democratic and personal, the kind of activity where you are more often riding against the clock and your own limitations than against other people. That is what makes cycling challenging, and everyone a champion. Carl H. Antczak, a gentleman who lost 200 pounds, writes, "I enjoy nothing better than being out on a back road, observing nature firsthand with nothing noisier than the clicking of my chain as it spins through my freewheel. Cycling gives me a great sense of accomplishment as I have achieved goals I never thought I was capable of five years ago."

William Melton of Rockville, Maryland, rides because it helps his arthritis, an injured rotator cup, and a broken right hip, now mending. He rides 3,500 miles a year to stay loose and to challenge himself mentally. Perhaps more than most he is able to ride long distances, even with pain, because he has mastered the skills needed to excel. Melton is another example of how cycling meets us at our level of need.

CADENCE

Pedal cadence is fundamental to successful cycling, yet few cyclists learn the science. Contrary to what might seem natural and even efficacious at first, you should pedal at a brisk 80 revolutions per minute, less on the hills, of course, and on demanding single tracks. Racers generally pedal in excess of 100 rpm, dropping to 70–80 spins for climbing. The rule of thumb is to pedal faster than might seem natural in the beginning, using a well-articulate range of gears to keep your cadence smooth. However, this is easier said than done. I recall visiting the Penn State University Biomechanics Lab a few years ago and was happy to have a computer record my cadence but not happy with the printout Dr. Peter Cavanaugh gave me. The computer showed that I attained peak pedal force at about 90°, or with the pedal at 3 o'clock. Significant downward pressure was still being recorded at the bottom of the stroke (180°, or 6 o'clock). Downward pressure decreases but is not eliminated during the upstroke, acting in opposition to the other leg.

For years cycling coaches have recommended that you pull on the upstroke, though all the research I've seen suggests few people, even elite cyclists, actually do this. The advice has consequences. The driving leg has the daunting task of lifting a 30–40-pound resting limb perhaps 100 times a minute. The best that most recreational and racing cyclists can hope for is to consciously think about pedaling in the "round," rather than in the square, to effectively unweigh the resting leg and lift the pedal slightly. Cyclists who have perfected this technique use only 70 percent as much force as those with the worst pedal strokes. Studies have shown that recreational cyclists improved their pedal strokes after an analysis similar to the one conducted on me at Penn State.

Most of us, however, are not hooked up to computers and must use our imagination. Some racers imagine themselves scraping mud from their shoes at the bottom of the stroke. Racer Alex Stieda likens pedaling action to walking on eggs. "I realize it's weird, but when you walk this way you drop your heel then push off with the ball of the foot. It's similar to the ankling effect. The idea is to keep it smooth and avoid mashing on the downstroke."

Stieda also tells riders to "pedal from the hip. I'll ride beside them and put my finger on their hipbone. Think of it as a pivot point. Hold it steady and let the legs turn circles."

These recommendations flow from the assumption that you are wearing equipment appropriate to the sport. I've decided to treat equipment needs within the context of cycling rather than list them as an expensive grab bag for the new cyclists to purchase. To be sure, you can cycle in anything and most people do. But if you are to be an efficient, effective cyclist, you'll need some kind of cycling shoes. You have some choices but make sure what you have is a cycling shoe with a stiff shank. The pedal is hard, and if you wear a running shoe, you'll feel it after a few miles.

At the very least I recommend you have toe clips on your bike as they will help keep your feet secure and permit you to concentrate on cadence. Please don't worry about toe clips tying you to the pedal; you can always pull out quickly, effortlessly, and safely.

Many companies offer touring, all-purpose mountain bike or fitness shoes which have the stiff shank but are still flexible enough to walk in. Avocet and Specialized make fine cycling shoes, and I can recommend them without hesitation.

As you become more involved in cycling, you might want to consider clipless pedals. The bottom of the cycling shoe locks into the pedal cage itself, permitting one to deliver much more power to the pedal stroke. The question recreational cyclists have about this system is: "How can I get my feet out in an emergency?" Easy—a twist to the side or a sharp pull will free you. Frankly, I was not enamored of this new technology when it was first introduced six years ago. I had

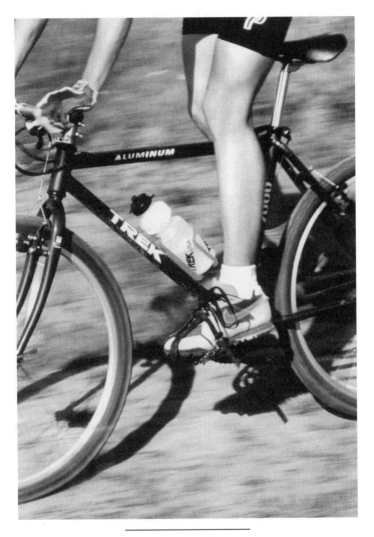

"Toe clips on your bike will help keep your feet secure and permit you to concentrate on cadence."

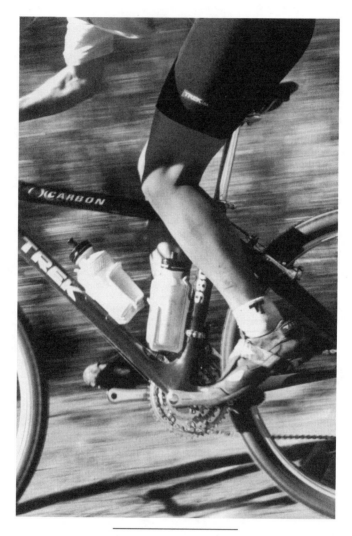

"On clipless pedals the bottom of the cycling shoes locks into the pedal cage itself, permitting one to deliver much more power to the stroke."

ridden tens of thousands of miles with my toe clips and straps and was quite happy. If I had not been shamed into changing to Shimano clipless by my staff, I might still be in the dark ages. I became an immediate convert. Not only did I fit my bike better—I wasn't sliding around on the pedals—but I felt stronger and certainly climbed hills better. I improved my cadence and my times.

When you are comfortable on the bike, know it like a good friend, and feel ready to go to the next level, I encourage you to fit the bike with clipless pedals. You can certainly become a very fit and healthy rider without them. However, why not make your time on the bike as efficient and comfortable as possible? I have no stock in these companies, but unabashedly recommend clipless pedals.

One caveat: Though clipless pedals are available for mountain bikes and have enthusiastic supporters, many mountain bikers prefer toeclips and straps, particularly for off-road riding that requires frequent starts, stops, dismounts, portages, and the like. Your bike-riding style and cycling terrain will dictate what's best for you. Since this book is not about log jumping or climbing Slickrock in Moab, Utah, I'm recommending equipment that will help you become a performance rider. In the long run, time in the saddle will be one gauge of fitness, and you might as well be comfortable and productive on your bike. I cannot emphasize cadence enough. Whether you are turning the pedals at 100 rpm or 60 rpm, you will have a certain rhythm to riding. A comfortable, even elegant rhythm comes from being on a lightweight, responsive bike with gearing appropriate to your power, physiology, and ambition. To bring "roundness" to this pedaling, some racers and enthusiasts ride a single-speed, direct drive (no freewheel) track bike which forces them to keep pedaling. Such practice is not completely esoteric. Within a few miles of my office is the Lehigh County Velodrome, a banked oval track, where a cross section of Rodale employees participate in skill-building clinics with particular emphasis on cadence. We all feel it makes us stronger, more efficient, and able to better concentrate on pedaling through bottom dead center of the stroke.

LIGHT RIDING

Top American professional Andy Hampsten has said that psychologically it's a boost to have a light bike, a fact that he repeats in his head like a mantra on a long climb. I, however, am no prophet of the "lightness is all" philosophy in cycling, which puts titanium in seat posts, stems, and handlebars, just to eliminate a few grams of weight. It makes more sense to lose that weight from the thighs and stomach.

Still, riding a bike that weighs 24 pounds will make a world of difference, particularly if you're used to riding one well over 30 pounds, the weight of many department store bikes. A light bike that fits moves when you command it. A light bike floats beneath you, adding to your comfort.

If I recommend that you ride a lightweight bike, I also suggest you ride lightly. I'm talking about how you "wear" your bike. You won't be able to ride lightly if the saddle is too low or high or too far forward, the most common problem associated with new cyclists. Try it. You'll discover it's not comfortable to have your saddle far forward because too much weight is put on your arms. Your arms and back get tired.

I have asked hundreds of amateurs and professional cyclists, including Tour de France winner Greg LeMond, for one piece of advice that applies to cyclists of all abilities. Most often the response is, "Relax on the bike." So let's begin with the hands.

Gripping the handlebars tightly will simply translate road shock up through your hands, arms, and neck. You'll feel every mile. Racers know to hold the bars lightly, steering rather than driving the bike. One advantage of the traditional drop handlebar is that you can move the hands around for comfort, leverage, and relief. For normal straight line cycling at 12–15 mph, well within the ability of a recreational cyclist, place the hands about 2 inches from either side of the stem. A narrower grip sacrifices leverage and control while a wider one increases wind drag. Keep your wrists and elbows slightly bent. Again, hold the bars lightly but keep a couple of fingers around the bar for safety. Greg LeMond suggests pulling up on the bars with one arm while pushing with the opposite leg, a technique useful on climbs.

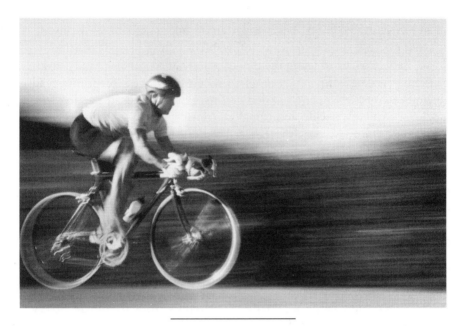

"One advantage of the traditional drop handlebar is that you can move the hands around for comfort, leverage, and relief."

To ride with one hand, a skill that is useful when you want to drink from the water bottle or just stretch, place the working hand an inch from the stem to avoid oversteering. But always check to make certain the pavement is smooth. A pothole could break your grip and send you sprawling.

To relax and slightly improve your aerodynamic position, put your hands on the brake hoods, the best place when riding on the flat or with a group. The thumbs are to the inside of the hood with one or two fingers on the levers for easy braking. The palms rest comfortably on the curves of the brake hoods.

Play with this position, finding what works for you. On a long ride, I find myself resting my palms on the hoods as one way to relieve pressure on my hands.

Though getting down on the drops on a road bike is the most

aerodynamic position, I use it for short bursts and occasionally descending. It's simply too uncomfortable for long periods of time.

The real secret to using the downturned handlebars is to fully utilize them, moving your hands often to relieve numbness or pressure. Of course, you are wearing padded cycling gloves and even padded handlebar tape to provide additional cushion.

Davis Phinney, much decorated American racer who operates a camp in Avon, Colorado, with his wife, ex-racer Connie Carpenter, reports that one thing most people coming to his training camp have in common is that they are rigid on a bike, holding it tight, using brakes rather than skills to move around obstructions or out of trouble.

I have been on many organized rides, some drawing up to 10,000 cyclists of different abilities, a state that is usually underscored by the horrible screech of thousands of brake pads as the throngs of cyclists descend even a modest grade. I've ridden in a pack with riders who cycle 100 miles without moving their hands from the brake hoods. Racers talk about feathering the brakes, using them softly, just enough to slow down. Learn to cycle out of difficult situations. When you must brake, do so gently. The front brake is the most powerful and useful, particularly when the road is good and dry. Otherwise, use the front and rear. Know your stopping distance on different surfaces in different weathers. The well-schooled cyclist tries to anticipate light changes, car door openings, horses on the trail, and responds accordingly. Remember you are indeed "lightness" perched on your bike, feathering your brakes, shifting smartly in subtle increments that answer the needs of your lungs and legs. Such behavior constitutes soft cycling and is within the grasp of everyone reading this book.

I consider cycling in its purest form to be play. Study children on BMX bikes who make any obstacle a playground. Elite cyclists have long accepted the "bump and dodge" drill as both a form of play and a way to be light and lighthearted in a pack. When comfortable on the bike, try this exercise. Find a partner of similar size to practice with. Mike Walden, coach of some of the greatest American cyclists of the last 40 years, recommends riding around a traffic-free course side by side at a steady pace. Bump elbows and shoulders while looking straight ahead. The secret is to keep your bike vertical while you lean into your partner. Stay relaxed and keep your elbows bent. Chances are if you bump into someone on a real ride, you'll remain loose.

Another drill that Coach Walden uses is to put 8–10 toilet plungers ten feet apart on a traffic-free road and have his students ride straight for the plungers, moving the bike quickly around them, first to one side, then the other. The key is to keep your body over the plunger while moving the bike beneath you. If you are really looking for a challenge, try the "bump and dodge" drills at the same time.

This play actually has very practical applications. I must have used this technique a thousand times to avoid glass, nails, dogs, cow dung, and the like. Mastering this technique is worth its weight in gold. Whatever the obstacle, the bike is always easier to control when it's under way. Skill is always your best ally, not brakes.

PACELINE RIDING

Most cyclists ride alone. However, you usually don't improve much if you don't cycle with people who can teach you a thing or two. I regularly ride with cyclists 20–30 years younger and by midseason can usually stay with them. In fact, I'm pleased if I still hold them in view after the first ten miles. My answer to the above dilemma is to ride by myself during the week and find some company on weekends.

If you are serious about cycling, you will find other cyclists, perhaps in your local cycling club. One way or another you will meet them on the road. After all, who else is out at 5 A.M. on a Sunday morning? So, whether with a few friends or a club, you will likely ride in a group and soon find the advantages to riding the paceline, that is, riding tightly behind each other, because it's the most efficient way to ride in a group at any speed. After all, paceline riding is fun and elegant, and it offers an energy savings of more than 25 percent.

Once on a ride, a paceline forms naturally with the stronger riders getting out front and the others tucked in behind, happy for the shelter. Except in races when there's a tactical advantage in not going to the front to take a pull, rarely do I see a recreational cyclist who won't in the spirit of fair play not take a turn at the front. Not surprisingly, cyclists have a natural fear of drafting or getting too close to the rider in front, due to the danger of overlapping wheels, a sure way to hit the pavement. The one bad spill I took some years ago occurred when I overlapped the wheel of the rider in front. I didn't follow my own advice.

Of course, you should avoid touching and overlapping wheels. Coach Walden had his students practice these actions, emphasizing that you should steer the bike, not lean and turn, when contact is made. Ask a friend to ride in front, in a straight line on a traffic-free road. Overlap his or her rear wheel slightly, simulate touching the wheel but immediately steer away without overcorrecting, the cause of most crashes and the reason I went down. Repeat this drill often and you'll become much more comfortable in the paceline.

You'll need a few cycling friends for this next drill. You'll need two pacelines of three or four riders cycling side by side on a safe stretch. The faster lane, on the left, is the advance line. Riders reaching the front swing off to the right, following into the relief line, eventually taking position at the end of the advance line, to begin the process over again. Care must be taken when swinging into the relief line, particularly if your group consists of novice cyclists.

When drafting, many riders stay too far behind their partner's rear wheel for fear of crashing. The key to a good draft is to continually make subtle adjustments to match the leader's pace. Rest your hands on the brake hoods or drops but try not to use the brakes. Instead of watching your partner's rear wheel, watch his whole bike, anticipating his next move. Look over or around him to see what's ahead. Try to stay within 6 inches of the leader's wheel. If you nudge closer, don't coast; rather, ease up on the pedals a bit. If you continue to close the gap, move a few inches to the left without overlapping wheels. Straighten your body. The wind will slow you.

I believe good pacelines come from familiarity. I am most comfortable sitting on the wheel of a friend or a cyclist I know fairly well. So find a group of cyclists with comparable abilities and get comfortable in the paceline. Whether you're cruising at 10 miles an hour or 20, you'll appreciate the company and discover how efficient paceline riding can be. One thing is for sure: It will enable you to stay on the bike longer and get the most out of your workout, central ingredients of a training program.

HILL CLIMBING

A friend of mind desperately seeks out cycling routes with no hills, a passion that almost cost us our friendship. I even cycled with him from Allentown, Pennsylvania, to Ocean City, Delaware, and back, the flattest course imaginable. Eventually I did get him to cycle across Pennsylvania and the length of Britain. But still the hills are anathema to him.

He's not unusual. Most cyclists avoid hills. Frankly, with the right bikes, technique, and attitude, I think you can learn to love the hills as I have done, seek them out, challenge them, defy them because hills can be a vital center of your cardiovascular conditioning program. When I want a quick barometer of my fitness, I head for the hills. You can too—and enjoy the ride.

Remember, if your bike has the right gearing for the terrain, there is no hill you can't climb. I think I can say that categorically about roads; I'm not so confident about off-road courses. I've encountered lots of hills I can't climb. But I keep trying. My point is that hills should not be feared. The secret is technique. Most cyclists wait far too long before downshifting. Think of a hill in three phases: the approach, the climb, and the crest. Whatever your pedal revolutions, once your cadence begins to drop off, however slightly, downshift immediately, and spin briefly at an unnaturally high rpm. The hill will quickly bring you back to your level. Apply this rule of thumb throughout the climb. When you reach the crest, don't coast. Pedal down the other side.

Whether one should be in or out of the saddle during climbing has caused heated debate. Often the hill decides. We know the Tour de France riders, who have to contend with the Alps and Pyrenees, sit 90 percent of the time. Rule of thumb: If the grade is steady and not too steep, try to stay in the saddle. Racers and hill climbers *par excellence*

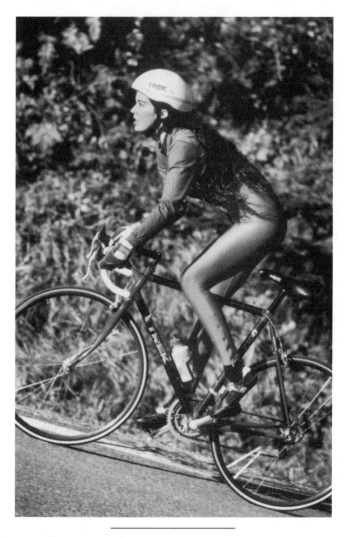

"Think of a hill in three phases: approach, climb, and crest."

recommend you stand in a slightly bigger gear and use the entire body to get over a steep patch. Once out of the saddle your caloric needs and heart rate go up.

Another key to successful out-of-saddle climbing is to make sure your body is in sync with your legs. Otherwise, too much swaying results in lost energy and puts you at risk. Here's how. Rest the V of your hands on the hoods, index and middle fingers around the bars. As you push down on the right pedal, pull up on the bar with the left hand. Let the bike rock but no more than a foot off-center.

Davis Phinney recommends not standing for too long because of additional oxygen consumption. When in good form, he'd stand for no more than a minute. But when tired, up to five minutes because it's the only way to get power to the pedals. For Phinney and for most cyclists, it's a matter of fitness. He tends to sit after a long tour, when he's stronger. You'll tend to sit after completing a century.

The temptation on a long torturous climb is to weave to cut the gradient. Sometimes it's necessary but usually a sign of being undertrained or overgeared. When I am forced to weave, I am very tired.

MORE CLIMBING TIPS

Here are twenty more climbing tips, courtesy of the *Bicycling* magazine editors.

1. Lighten your bike.
2. Lighten yourself.
3. Inflate your tires to maximum pressure.
4. Reduce wind resistance.
5. Start in lower gears.
6. Shift up when you stand.
7. Sit 90 percent of the time.
8. Scorn big gears.
9. Grip the brake hoods.
10. Grip the handlebars lightly.
11. Sway when standing.

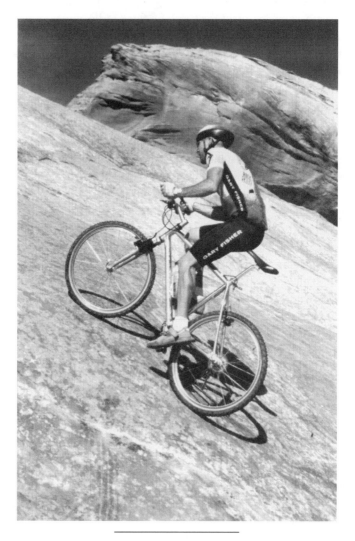

"Racers and hill climbers recommend you stand in a slightly bigger gear and use the entire body to get over a steep patch."

12. Shift before a hill.
13. Don't bounce your body.
14. Blend breathing/climbing.
15. Ride in a straight line.
16. Ride in front of a group.
17. Watch climbers on TV.
18. Check saddle height.
19. Relax the shoulders.
20. Do it again.

CORNERING

Most cyclists tend to slow down, squeeze the brakes, and stop pedaling when they come to a corner. Even for the professionals, this section is the most dangerous, where crashes and pileups occur. In tight, closed-circuit races such as criteriums, corners always draw the biggest crowds.

Whether you are taking the corner with 120 professional racers or with friends on a Sunday afternoon, the advice is the same: relax. Remember the "bump and dodge" drill? Well, corners are where you get the most bumping and dodging and require your most relaxed state.

As you approach a corner, put your hands on the drop bars in a relaxed manner. Move your weight back slightly so you can steer from the rear of the saddle. Keep the inside pedal up to prevent it from hitting the road. Straighten the outside leg and push down. Look ahead of the bike in front. Brake slightly before the turns. Canadian professional Alex Stieda suggests you start as far to the outside as possible, out to the apex, then go in wide as conditions permit. Lean your body and bike as you round the corner. If you are more ambitious, you might try overbanking, a technique recommended by many professionals. It involves leaning the bike a lot and keeping the body upright. Overbanking is best suited for tight turns in dry conditions. Simply, you lean into the corner by countersteering, turning the bar for a second in the opposite direction from where you want to go.

Once angled properly, steer back into turn. Lean your bike more than in the first example, straightening your inside arm and pressing on the bar with the inside hand, making your torso move upright.

Fred Zahradnik, *Bicycling* editor, reports learning the technique of overbanking at the Phinney camp. "Our preliminary overbanking practice took place on a slalom course in a parking lot. You can set up a similar one on an empty lot some Sunday morning. Cones are best for marking the turns, but lacking these, the intersection of parking lines, about 30 feet apart, will work."

Whichever way you come through a corner, remember the cornering IOUs. When coasting through a turn, keep the *inside* pedal up, keep weight on the *outside* pedal, and keep your head *up*.

Although some of the above tips will carry over into your off-road riding, there are some differences when cornering on dirt. You'll want to approach the turn wide, moving to the inside as you cross the turn, and move wide again. As with your road bike, you'll want to brake before the turn. Because you may catch a pedal on a rock or downed tree, keep the cranks horizontal. Likewise you'll want to lean into the turn while pushing down on the outside pedal. If you seem to be going too wide, let the inside leg or arm flutter a little to help the line through. Then, put some power to the pedals.

The more off-road riding you do, the more skilled you'll become on the road. These are complementary activities. Let them teach each other a lesson.

MOUNTAIN BIKE CADENCE

Almost all research associated with pedaling has come in through the road bike door, and even though the new breed of mountain bikers often looks askance at the road bike rider, they might learn something from the latter, especially when it comes to spinning, a skill mountain bikers don't take seriously. Spinning means pedaling both faster and better.

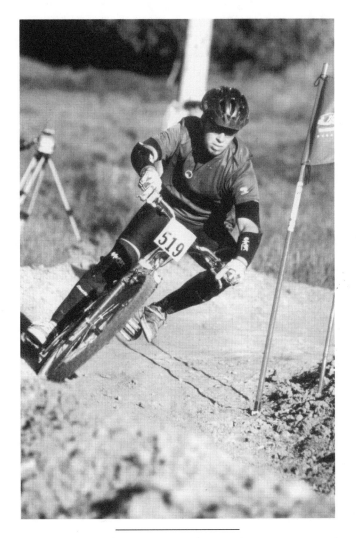

"Approach the turn wide, moving to the inside as you cross the turn, and move wide again."

JAMES C. McCULLAGH

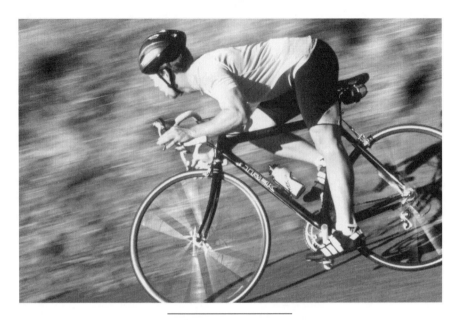

"For fast descending on the road, drop your torso to keep the center of gravity low."

DESCENDING

From my observations, most mountain bikes, or perhaps more correctly, cyclists on mountain bikes, like other cyclists, tend to chop at, stomp on, and push down on the pedals usually at a relatively low rpm, which is significantly affected by terrain and gearing—we always come back to that. I don't know why mountain bikers seem more prone to stomping on the pedals. My guess is that rather than rejecting the elegance of a road rider, they really believe they are hiking, in the woods and all, one foot in front of the other.

To curb the habit of hiking, stomping, or romping on the pedals, listen to the road rider:

1. Push down.
2. Before the pedal reaches bottom, pull back on it as if trying to scrape mud off a shoe.
3. Pull up.
4. Before the pedal reaches the apex, push forward.

You can go fast and still be safe on descents. Here's how.

1. Place your hands on the drops but in reach of the brakes.
2. Pedal softly to prevent lactic acid buildup.
3. Shift your weight rearward on the saddle.
4. Drop your torso to keep the center of gravity low.
5. Grip brakes lightly to moderate speed. To slow, raise your chest into the wind.
6. Look far ahead.

By concentrating on the dynamics of pedaling, you'll become a smoother, faster pedaler. There's a lot of debate about optimal cadence for mountain bikes. My rule of thumb is that if you fall below 40 rpm on a climb, you probably need lower gears. A final rule of thumb from the road: If your lungs are fatigued, slow your cadence. If your legs hurt, speed up.

OFF-ROAD SKILLS

Although the skill you need to be a good road rider will contribute to your off-road riding ability, the two sports have enough differences that they warrant separate treatment. By becoming equally skilled in both activities, you'll be better prepared for a full, year-round, all-season cycling program. Incidentally, don't listen to the cyclists who will put you in different camps, segregated like bivouacking armies. Road and off-road riding are complementary activities. The 2 million readers of *Bicycling* magazine get better doing both, spending more time on the bike in the process. You can too. More to the point: Ned Overend, mountain bike world champion, rides his road bike for 1.5 hours of light spinning on the flats after a hard Sunday race. The important thing is to spend time in the saddle, to enjoy the experience, and to keep moving, not the kind of bike you ride. You'll find your vehicle of choice. I want to make sure you use it.

From the inception, the road bike was an instrument of speed. Bike races against the clock, horses, and trains were not uncommon at the turn of the last century. In the 1970s and 1980s, however, hundreds of thousands discovered the pleasant, peripatetic crawl of the touring bike—a longer version of the traditional road bike described here—because the road bike had taken the form of its European cousin. For most, this bike means speed, racing, and performance. For the layperson, it means fast recreational riding.

The mountain bike, hatched in the hands and heads of colleagues and friends in northern California and Colorado fifteen years ago, has had a much different puberty, more raucous, more youthful, though perhaps not more daring than growing up on the road. To be sure, the 30,000 licensed mountain bike racers, particularly those who specialize in downhill events, believe they invented speed. But the sport is really in the hands of the millions who use these fat, sturdy, nearly trouble-free bikes for pleasure or just getting around. And they know, as my research has shown, that fitness is always waiting at the back door. When I ride a mountain bike, I think of dirt, tracks, the environment, and limbs that leave welts on my face as I try to duck under, at speed, another spreading chestnut tree.

I live on a small farm in eastern Pennsylvania. I like riding on my farm for sheer play. I can fall down, jump over logs (and fail), take a header (with helmet) on a soft path as I practice my unruly descents, and get a most deserved mud bath as I cycle through a patch infested with spring. Moreover, I can do all this and still be an insignificant part of the landscape. I am not exaggerating to say a barred owl talks to me as I cycle softly in the early evening on the edge of the nesting area. I answer, of course.

Perhaps mountain biking invited metaphor because the context one moves through changes both radically and subtly, demanding comparisons and a rich texture of language to match the rich vocabulary of the sport.

Let me repeat myself. No more than 18 percent of the more than 6 million mountain bikes sold last year ever find the dirt. Most are ridden on streets, bike and canal paths, and in parks which, though all virtuous activities, are not what this beast was designed to do. The mountain bike is designed for the off-road, to be ridden hard. And that activity requires skills not found in the road bike handbook.

FINDING A LINE

When shopping for a mountain bike, you'll find a lot with front and rear suspension—you know, shock absorbers. Of the mountain bikes on the market as you read this book, 30 percent will have front suspension and 10 percent both front and rear. And these numbers are growing by the year as manufacturers are finally understanding that bicycles are not motorcycles and are designing suspension systems that are lightweight and functional. I ride bikes without suspension systems, and with front and rear suspension. Certainly when I ride a washboard single track that makes my teeth chatter so much I feel I have dentures, a suspended bike is a blessing. On the other hand, when I'm riding a steep, rock-strewn single track, I can do without the weight. Please keep in mind that while suspension serves useful psychological and mechanical ends—*Bicycling* magazine has done the test to confirm their value—most beginners, cyclists who stick to the roads, and those with no intention of going off-road, don't need a bike with suspension. The terrain will dictate. I know cyclists who use a front suspended bike for commuting because the roads in their town are so bad they feel as if they're cycling through a mine field. We'll meet others later on who use suspended bikes to combat back injuries.

A bike without suspension is especially suited to helping you become a skillful rider. To a degree, you want to feel the bike beneath you. My editors who ride everything of consequence on the market have said more than once: Suspension not only absorbs road shock, but absorbs one's mistakes. One of the first things you learn about trail or single-track riding is finding a line. Essentially that means you pick a line through a trail, stream, or muddy patch and stay with it. As you travel, you make minor adjustments depending on your reading of the terrain. If you pick a line through inhospitable rocks, you will know it soon enough, through the shock transferred up your arms or by falling. One reason cyclists like suspension is that the technology gobbles up that rough patch. Without the suspension crutch—and it's often that for beginners—you must be more attuned to your surrounding, watching the trail for slight irregularities. You learn to ride a good line by riding a good line, hoping all the time the hand-eye coordination your parents gave you is up to the task. I've learned more by stopping, starting, falling, climbing back in the saddle, and riding a hill till I get it right than by riding a dual suspension limousine.

When I first rode a mountain bike in Crested Butte, Colorado, trying to climb 15 percent grades and thundering, often out of control, down precipitous single tracks, I received an early lesson. Mountain biking is not about power or muscles or ability to push a big gear; it's about skill. I have seen the well-muscled, fit cyclists take a run at the legendary Slickrock, a steep sandstone rock on Moab, Utah, only to be disappointed, precisely because they depend on power, not skill. And they don't take the time to inspect the surface and find the almost imperceptible curves that offer a line up this stone challenge. Once visitors find the line buried discreetly in this ancient rock, they have much more success on the slippery slope.

Your fitness and health will be enhanced by your riding skills. As in any sport, skill is born of relaxation, precisely the habit most mountain bikers don't display. When you are relaxed, not only are you sitting softly and surely on the bike, ready for changes in terrain, but your vision is also relaxed, enabling you to see beyond the front wheel. I learned early following a hard-riding, skillful woman along some tricky single tracks in Crested Butte that my bike did indeed follow my eyes. That's probably why I stumbled and fell so much. A novice, I fixed my stare on the front wheel or a bike length ahead, hoping to avoid obstacles. Doesn't work. Sure one has to be focused so as to not hang the pedal at 6 o'clock when going through a rock-strewn section of the trail. You need "near" vision and concentration to avoid obstacles at hand. But the key is to look and think seven or eight bike lengths ahead, imagining where the bike will be. That is "far" vision that will enable you to anticipate problems, consider any changes in the texture of the trail, think about the tree line that seems to be intersecting the trail in the distance. Beginners tend to fixate on the front wheel; skilled mountain bikers look and think 40–50 feet ahead, more on a downhill.

Off-road riders talk about "cleaning" a hill, a section, or a stream, meaning accomplishing the ride without putting a foot down, the brake often used when skill is lacking. Developing a "far" vision will enable you to pick a good line and negotiate a down tree but will also help you anticipate the rocks and stream ahead. The name of this game is anticipation.

Try a few simple exercises. Ride a trail with your eyes focused on your front wheel or slightly ahead. Chances are you will be gripping the handlebars tightly, waiting for the next bump. Now, with the front wheel within your gaze, take a broader, wider view, concentrating on the scene 40 feet ahead. You'll feel more like a tactician than a foot soldier, anticipating changes in the terrain, using your arms and legs naturally to induce a more comfortable ride. Far vision allows you to sit on the bike softly, torso steady, fingers resting lightly on the brake levers.

When beginning your off-road riding, stop often, take in the sights. Take in the trail ahead. Close your eyes, visualize the peaks and valleys, the rocks and debris. This is what athletes do through visualization techniques. Imagine yourself cycling softly and successfully through that section of trail, your line perfect, your body in control. Now do it, but open your eyes first.

Off-road riders talk about floating, and it feels just the way it sounds. When the bike traverses the trail marked by cambers, jagged edges, and inclines, the bike bounces. How much it bounces depends on the width of the tires and the air pressure. But the bounce and what shock is not absorbed by the tires (or a suspension system) will find its way up your legs, arms, and into your seat. How you receive that shock is the question. If you are relaxed, using your body as an intricate suspension system, you'll have a smoother, more comfortable ride. To do this, you must counter the movement a rough trail translates to the bike, especially the bottom bracket. Your arms and legs are the elastic which must counter this movement as the bike bounces. To be successful, you must be out of the saddle; otherwise, every time the bike bounces, your body will follow suit. By being out of the saddle, you can avoid literally bouncing around, effectively using your limbs as springs. The goal is to always keep the torso stable and your center of gravity concentrated. This way you'll be able to ride a good line and clean any section.

THE ART OF DESCENDING

The essence of mountain biking is sitting softly on the bike while skillfully taking in the terrain. Successful off-road riders are centered.

Veteran racer Jacquie Phelan remarked, "You can't ride and think about dinner or divorce or the bills. You need to be one big sensory receptor if you're going to stay within the margins of control. You need to be like an animal. They don't think about bills." And these remarks came after Jacquie, absentmindedly letting her foot rest in the 6 o'clock pedal position, caught a five-inch rock and went down.

Penny Davidson, national downhill champion, said this after taking a spill: "I didn't give the trail the respect it deserved. You should never get on a course without being focused."

The best mountain bikers are minimalists. One of my most memorable lessons I received from Hank Barlow, who really does float on his bike. I was in Crested Butte doing a piece for *Good Morning America* and Hank was the local talent, showing us spots for filming. He showed me more than that, particularly in climbing and descending. A beginner, I had the novice's fear of descending some of those cliffs at 11,000 feet, using my brakes as a weapon rather than a tool, following his line without grace or confidence. The squeal of my brakes, my stopping, starting, and cursing did not make the breakfast show but are indelible reminders to me that off-road riding is about grace, skill, and using the bike minimally. And nowhere is the minimalist art in greater demand than in braking and descending.

A comfortable position on the bike includes a comfortable position for the hands. To begin, find a favorite hand position. This might mean wrapping thumb and forefinger around handlebars and using the other fingers for braking. Others put their index, middle, and ring fingers on the levers. Choose a position that suits you. Even though brakes are often overused, they are still used. Keep them within reach.

Veterans suggest the number of fingers placed on the lever vary with the terrain, because some surfaces demand more handlebar control. For sand, gravel, and other soft stuff, try no fingers on the front brake and three on the rear. If you brake hard in front on these surfaces, you'll likely bog down. For steep descent, go with three fingers on each brake. Use a system that suits your bike and riding style.

Try to use the entire body when you brake. For example, slide your butt back in the saddle and grip the seat with your thighs. Involving your full body will help your braking and control.

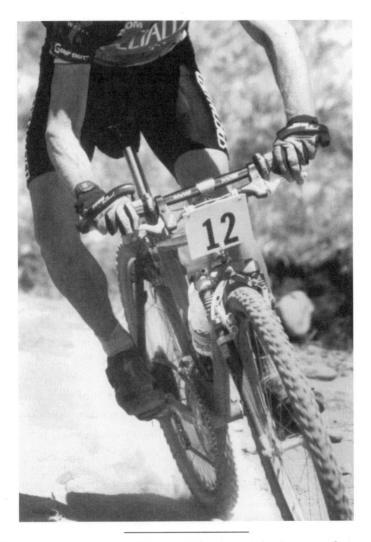

"Choose a position that suits you. Even though brakes are often over-used, they are still used. Keep them within reach."

Most off-road riders will become more efficient riders if they use their brakes less. Here are a few drills *Bicycling* magazine has suggested to help give up the habit.

○ 1. *Nonstop Drill* Find an open, empty, deserted spot, such as a parking lot, and get to know your bike. Play. Imagine you left the brakes at home. Explore ways to stop without brakes such as turning the front wheel, lifting it off the ground. Play with your center of gravity. Move around on the bike, through the bike, and watch what happens to your movement. Use your body as a brake.

○ 2. *Brakeless Drill* Leave the parking lot and go to a flat or slightly rolling single track. Make sure there are obstacles. The brakes are still at home. Feel how your bike moves over and through obstacles at speed. Practice shifts in balance to compensate for changes in speed. Practice cornering. Note how the unbraked bike finds its way through a corner.

○ 3. *Hill Drill* Brakes are still at home. Find a single track with small hills, nothing steep enough to invite despair. Stay under 15 mph on the descents. You want to be going fast enough to worry so concentrate on the field of vision, the rhythm of the ride. Let the bike take you along. Feel the flow. If you want to slow down, use your body and the bike, not the brakes.

○ 4. *Hillier Drill* Brakes are still at home. Go to the top of a steep single track and descend without hitting the brakes. If you cheat, you still win. Minimizing the use of brakes will allow you to concentrate on the ride.

Descending is an art, not a science. The tendency for most cyclists is to ride the brakes down a hill, causing havoc to the trail surface and possible injury to the rider. The scene is familiar. Your heart sinks when you crest a hill and see a monster descent staring you in the face. Likely as not, if a rider does not skid his or her way to the bottom, he will take a tumble some-where along the way. That can be avoided. Here's how.

a. *Start slow.* Gonzo riders will rave about daredevil descents down technical hills. That's not me and probably not you. Better to start slow and accelerate under control.
b. *Slide back on the saddle.* The steeper the descent, the farther you should move back. This move adjusts your center of gravity.
c. *Stay behind the front brake.* It's the most powerful so use it, but with discretion. Too hard and you'll flip over the handlebars. Use the rear brake lightly to prevent the wheel locking.
d. *Go with the flow.* Momentum will get you through most obstacles so let it take you. Get your front wheel through, and the rear wheel will follow.
e. *Take some pressure out of your tires.* This will increase traction and help keep the bike upright at slow speeds when you descend.
f. *Walk if the descent seems too tricky or steep.* Better to dismount at the top rather than halfway down. Veteran riders do this all the time. I have walked on numerous occasions.

I have a steep single track within easy distance of my home and I go there to practice my descents. Some days I'll spend hours just trying to get them right, experimenting with moving back in the saddle and using minimal braking. Trees, rocks, and an occasional Doberman get in my way. I have ridden the course a hundred times and still fall, though I usually have the presence of mind to fall in the softest spot. The point is I learn something each time and get a little better. I learn the surfaces, knowing my bike responds differently to wet leaves than to snow. One fall reminded me of a remark made by John Tomac, one of the sport's best racers: "Don't treat snow patches like grass. Use good judgment, and don't take unnecessary chances." Good advice from a wily veteran who knows something about descents. He was going 40 mph when he hit a snow patch in the Sierra Mountains and slid 150 feet.

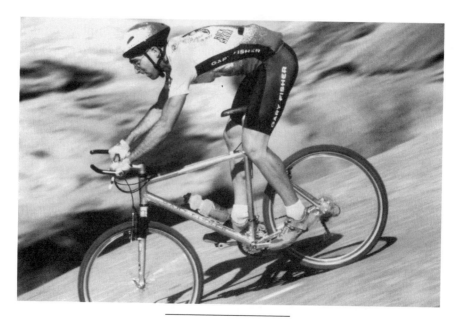

"The steeper the descent, the farther you should move back on the saddle."

CLIMBING WITHIN YOUR POWER

As I write this, I look out on my farm meadow covered with twenty inches of snow. With my eyes I can trace the single tracks and almost remember all the rocks, cambers, tree limbs, deer droppings, and dead moles along the way. I can see clearly a sharp line along the ridge where the barred owl nests, a single track that is really a staggered, three-piece climb with a sharp switchback. It has taught me a lot about climbing.

Most of us believe that one's ability to climb is directly related to the power put to the pedals. Therefore, it's not uncommon to see a cyclist roaring down one hill and pedaling furiously to get up the next, becoming confused when his momentum gives out and he's left wondering what to do in the middle of the hill. Though power properly

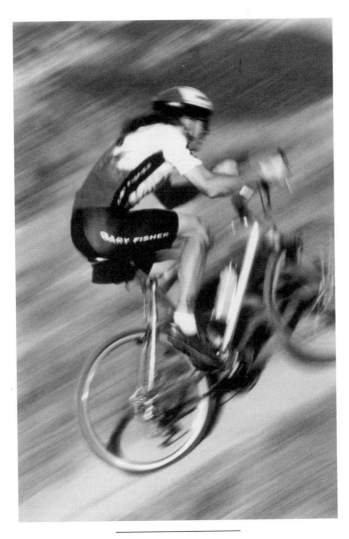

"Maintain momentum so you can get up the first part of the climb but not so much that the bike is bounced around by changes in the terrain."

applied is a definite advantage, off-road cycling is not a power game, and one can say that in spades about hill climbing. Cyclists have called this condition climbing within range or climbing at the edge of power, the latter having more poetry because it invites picturing oneself perched on the edge of the saddle, responding to incremental changes in terrain.

Climbing on the edge of power really is about that fine line between holding the line and losing traction, something every off-road rider has experienced. Too much power, and you lose it. Too little, and you stall and fall, especially if you are negotiating loose gravel. Ideally you become the equilibrist, balanced just right, holding traction delicately.

Here are some things to remember as you go into a climb:

1. Maintain sufficient momentum so you can get up the first part of the climb but not so much that the bike is bounced around by changes in the terrain.
2. Anticipate terrain changes and be in the right gear when you need it. You can't power up an off-road climb as you can on the road.
3. Ride the hill as slowly as possible, maintaining enough momentum that you won't fall.
4. Use your lowest gears.
5. Pull down and back on the handlebars, countering the thrust of the pedals, thus helping to control tire slippage.
6. Get out of the saddle and stay low with your buttocks slightly above the seat.
7. Keep side-to-side movement to a minimum with your torso steady.
8. Look for slight depressions on the uphill so you can relax and perhaps let the bike coast for a second or two.
9. Shift your body forward to keep the front wheel on the ground.
10. If you don't clean a hill the first time, go back and try again. I do it all the time.

OBSTACLE COURSE

If off-road riding were all ups and downs, life would be simple indeed. Unfortunately, Mother Nature intervenes and provides mud, rocks, sand, bumps, and more magnificent compression to delight the mountain biker. To get you around this pleasure circuit, here's some advice.

1. Mud. Mud is nothing to play with, so when you have a choice, stay away. But if you can't, at least be prepared.

Watch the trail for the inhospitable dirt-to-mud transition, braking before you hit the goo, gearing down, and sliding slightly forward. Try to pick a straight line and maintain some momentum. Pedal lightly.

Sometimes good sense and environmental ethics dictate that you get off and walk. Be wary of muddy slopes that "flow" into a stream. Riding these will definitely cause erosion.

Remember that the least damaging line through a mud hole is the center. Most people do the opposite and ride around the edges, making the pond bigger and perhaps contributing to erosion. One of the pleasures of the sport is getting muddy; don't miss it.

2. Sand. If you live in or near the desert, get really wide tires and keep them underinflated, around 30–40 psi. As with mud, the idea is to keep going, which means pointing your bike straight ahead. Any turns will surely stop you. Try and position your weight equally between the front and rear wheel. Too much weight either way and the respective wheels will bog down. If you begin to slow down, downshift to maintain acceleration. Move your weight back, drop your elbow, and pull down on the bars. If you start to lose momentum on an uphill, it is best to get off and walk.

3. Rocks. You can't be timid entering a rock garden. You'll be bounced around a lot so get out of the saddle and use arms and legs for shock absorption. Balance the weight on the balls of your feet, bend the knees, and grip the handlebars firmly. Pick the right line, but since rocks have legs and move around, be ready to improvise. Stay

75

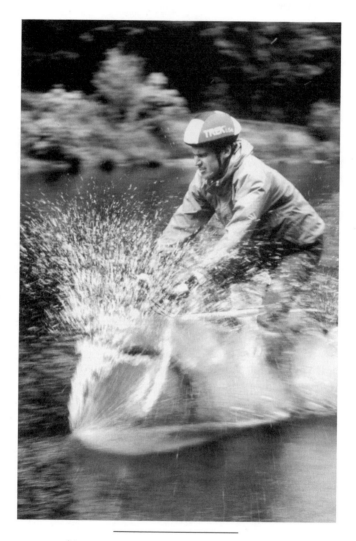

"When approaching a stream, pick a direct line and beware of the conditions and depth of the water."

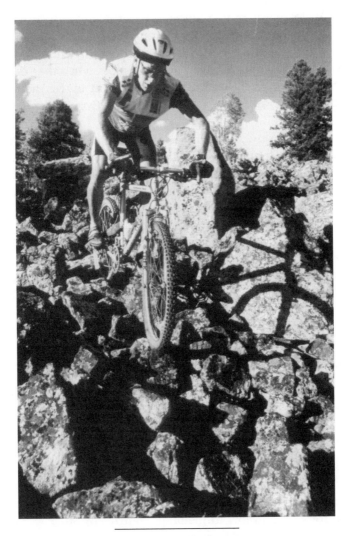

"To ride through a rock field, get out of the saddle and use arms and legs for shock absorption."

light and ready, maintaining momentum at all costs. Be in a gear that allows you to power over obstacles. If you do hit a rock with your pedal, don't panic, just lean away from it while staying out of the saddle. Sometimes the passage is so narrow that you must employ half-pedal strokes but that's a rarity for most. On other occasions, you'll have to ride right over a rock. Simply lift up on the bars and push the bike forward with a powerful pedal stroke.

4. Channels. A groove, a channel, a rut; whatever you call it, the beast can swallow your bike. Some cyclists tend to brake hard when entering a groove or a deep channel that's hard to get through. The result is skidding, which is not good for the cyclist or the terrain. Others propose speed. Still others suggest a technique called weaving. Before entering a groove, moderate your speed, slide back on the saddle, touch the brakes lightly, and start the weave, moving to opposite sides of the bank as you wind your way down a groove. Turn the bike with the handlebars and do not be leaning. Keep the pedals in a horizontal position as you brush the banks of the groove. You've just cleaned another piece of tricky terrain.

5. Bumps. Compressions, bumps, ruts, and any other configuration that changes the single track surface are likely to change your relationship with your bike, for the worse. But a little preparation can change the outcome. As is frequently the case, speed is the operative factor. You'll feel a bump or compression much more at high speed than low. So in the interest of safety, slow before you enter a compression, feathering the brakes. You want to be out of the saddle, weight back, pedals at the horizontal, arms and legs slightly flexed anticipating the front wheel hitting the depression. Let go of the brake levers as you hit. Be ready to begin a power stroke to move you out of the compression. Be forward and low to maintain control. In other words, float through this big hole in the trail.

6. Obstacles. *Mountain Bike* magazine's skills editor, known to all his fans as Captain Dondo, offers these suggestions for those who want to hop over obstacles such as logs. Approach the object at moderate

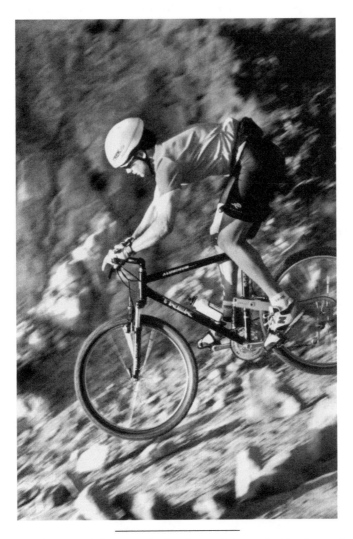

"Get out of the saddle, weight back, pedals at the horizontal, arms and legs slightly flexed, anticipating the front wheel hitting the depression."

speed, picking a takeoff point three feet in front. Compress your body in a catlike manner, arms and legs bent, ready to pounce. Launch your bike, front end first, pulling up on the handlebars. Twist the handlebar grips forward to help lift the rear wheel. Pull up with knees and feet to gain height. Fly. Touch down with both wheels and counter the impact of the landing with elbows, knees, and back.

By now you should indeed be flying. With a lightweight bike under you and the skills to handle the most challenging terrain, you are ready to make the bike a central part of your health, fitness, and training. You will become more skillful as you ride. In turn, your fitness will improve and your training will be pleasurable. For to be truly skillful on a bike is to be a dancer, a gymnast on a balance beam. To float is to be on the bike but above it, moving through the atmosphere at will. To be one with the bike is to feel the music as you ride. This symphony of the ride has as much to do with your spiritual well-being as your physical state.

I am reminded of Jack Chamberlin of San Diego, who suffered from the debilitating effects of drugs and alcohol before he took up mountain biking. "I find great joy and spiritual renewal in the *Geist* [spirit] of mountain biking," he reports. For Jack, cycling was the magical activity that helped him find the child within and made him whole again.

I can't tell you how many hundreds of people have touched me with similar stories. Sure, skills and techniques will make you a better rider and make your cycling more enjoyable. But I have a special spot in my heart for the people who drag their bikes out of the basement because their lives depend on it. Such a person is Geneva McMann of Auburn, Alabama, who has suffered from depression all her life. But while family members are on Prozac, she finds her therapy on mountain bikes. "I use [my bike] to maintain my self-esteem, to maintain my figure, and to maintain a 'no-depression' lifestyle. I outgrew my mountain bike and now have a new mountain and road bike. I ride between 110 and 150 miles per week. I pedal to feel good, to feel strong, to feel worthy. I can start a ride feeling low and twenty miles later I feel accomplished. I feel love, I feel like, I can love myself. As long as I stay on my bike, I know in my heart I will never fall back into old patterns. I long to ride, I crave it like a sweet. I will ride for the rest of my life. I will ride my bike to truly live and to truly love myself, which two years ago I couldn't love at all."

When you figure out how to jump logs and handle compression, when you can clean Slickrock with the best, I hope your heart resonates with the fundamental call of cycling, to make one whole again.

MOUNTAIN BIKE GEARING

Most mountain bikes have three chainrings in front and seven cogs or sprockets in the back. Count yours; simple math says that $3 \times 7 = 21$ gears. Right? Wrong! The reason for this condition is twofold. First, there is duplication in gearing. Second, certain gears require you to put your chain at an excessive angle and therefore are essentially useless. Let's say the low gear on my Barracuda mountain bike is 24 × 30T, which means the chainring in front has 30 teeth. That translates into a low gear of 20.8 inches, using the formula in the Appendixes. Try it on your bike.

Now, if I keep the chain on the 24T ring and move it to the third largest cog, say 20 percent, I'm in a 31.2-inch gear. If I shift to the middle chainring, say 36 percent, and back to the largest cog, 30T, I'm still in a 31.2-inch gear. That's what I mean by duplication. If you have the patience and stamina, try to resolve this before you leave the showroom floor. At least get a commitment from the shop that you can return, after riding the bike for a few weeks, to replace some cogs if necessary, at minimal or no cost.

The other reason you don't have 21 gears is that the chainline works best when it's parallel to the bike's straight line movement, such as when it's in the middle ring and middle cog. Stand behind the bike to confirm this. Now shift to the smallest ring and smallest cog. Note the slant in the chain. That gear is practically useless. If you did use it, you'd cause excessive wear to chain, cogs, and rings and be terribly put off by the clatter.

You might encounter this condition on other bikes, but since mountain bikes are the most popular products on the market and there's a lot of hype about their features, including gearing, I use this bike as an example. Again, a badly geared bike will affect cadence, comfort, hill climbing, and progress. In other words, every aspect of your cycling. Don't let it boggle you. Don't let the salesman confuse you. Above all, don't believe the story that high gears make the man or woman.

C·H·A·P·T·E·R F·I·V·E

BASIC TRAINING

In the past when I'd think of basic training, I'd think of Coach Scho-field at Taylor Alderdice High School in Pittsburgh, who was furious with me if I didn't vomit after an 880-yard race. Or my Texan com-pany commander at the Great Lakes Naval Center in Chicago, who, as punishment, made me climb rope until my hands were raw and bleed-ing. Now I think of tough bike climbs as challenge and adventure, the chance to do a century ride a blessing.

I must sound as if I'm middle-aged. Well, I am, but that's not the reason for my optimism. I am pleased that I can ride with men and women twenty and thirty years younger and still be competitive. I am pleased for the essential grace of mobility. Few days go by that I don't receive a letter from someone who has used the bike to come back to health. By comparison, I am appalled at my lack of resolve.

My mantra is this: Cycling meets you at your level of need. Joe Luna of Turlock, California, told me he was shot at point-blank range by a .357 Magnum when he tried to help someone in trouble. The bullet pierced his right side, cracked a rib, punctured a lung, and damaged his pelvis. The doctors thought he was going to die. He didn't. Once out of the hospital, he purchased a 40-pound Sears bike. Within a few years he was cycling 7,000 miles annually and to date has ridden more than 50,000 miles since his accident. He credits his complete recovery to bicycle riding.

Joe Luna went from the Intensive Care Unit to becoming a cycling enthusiast, fighting for his life in the process. His longest ride was from Carmel, California, to the Mexican border. Gayle Horowitz, of Flushing, New York, suffers from asthma and severe joint problems and writes, almost defiantly, "I am not ready to stop fighting yet and I'm not giving up my bike. As long as I can get on a bike and complete a pedal revolution, I will."

That is indeed basic training: completing a pedal revolution, a fundamental act of health and defiance. Though I will remind you throughout this book of "everyday heroes," people I am honored to mention, the task of motivating training, and keeping ourselves healthy is much simpler for most of us. We start with a turning of the pedal.

There is no perfect training schedule, no one program that suits all, no final piece of advice. Your training depends on your level of fitness, set of objectives, and lifestyle. Ask a hundred people for their training schedules, and you'll get a hundred different programs.

Take the schedule of Caroline Sandow of Tampa, Florida, who rides every day. First day, interval training; second, speed work; third, climbing; fourth, endurance (long ride); fifth, racing; sixth, technique; seventh, active rest ride. Phew. Her regimen would put many Olympians to shame.

Or Tim Mahaffey of Huber Heights, Ohio, who trains seriously during April and May, 70–100 miles a week. During June through August he usually does a coast-to-coast ride, having completed at least fourteen to date. He has ridden in forty-nine states. In the winter he slows down a bit, but not much.

Or Sam Amos of Kettering, Ohio, a self-proclaimed tourist who cycles over 3000 miles a year at an average speed of 13 miles per hour, often in a very low, granny gear (46X24T).

Or Dick Anderwald of Yakima, Washington, who begins training in "late winter/early spring with weekend training rides averaging 20–30 miles with a coffee and pancake stop at the halfway point. As the weather warms, I add two or three early morning weekday rides of 17 miles, which I try to finish in one hour. By April 15, the weekend miles have lengthened to 50–55 miles." By June, he is riding centuries. He rides a mountain bike for a change of pace. And now he rides a tandem so his youngest daughter can keep the pace.

And so on. My point is that training schedules are as varied as the people who follow them. To be successful, a schedule must be flexible, take into consideration other life needs, and contain a sizable element of rest and play. However, this doesn't mean your training should not have a recognizable structure and that you shouldn't monitor your progress. Quite the contrary. The more aware you are concerning the effects of training on your body, the better the cyclist you'll be. And you'll be much easier to live with.

I write this early in the morning, shut in by yet another blizzard that has ravaged the weary East. Of course I'm disappointed that the snow has cut into my bicycle commuting, though I'm pleased to get all this experience riding a mountain bike in snow. Still I'm ecstatic because I'm dreaming of a cycling trip across the South of France I'll take in six months. Maps cover my office walls with all arrows pointing to the wine regions. But I like the mountains and Brittany and the coast.

This dream will get me through my hour on the exercise bike and remind me that I have work to do. A trip of at least 1,000 miles requires some preparation, not the least of which is time in the saddle. If my long-term goal is to cycle across the South of France, my short-term goal is to get out on the roads and single tracks again, relearning the sport. I'll keep my long-range goal in mind but spend the next two or three months preparing a foundation. That is, easy miles in low gears. I don't care whether you are a racer or a fitness rider, whether off-road or on, when you move from a maintenance schedule to a training schedule, you have to take it slow and easy, putting in the base miles, building power and endurance.

This foundation building is the hardest lesson for most of us to learn. It's early spring, our legs are coming back, and we feel like flying. However, neither our legs or lungs are likely ready for the adventure. Restraint is not always easy. I have to force myself to stay out of the big chainring, whether on my mountain or road bike, until I have a thousand spring miles under my belt.

To get maximum health and fitness from your cycling will mean time in the saddle. How you spend that time is as important as how many miles you chalk up. Until quite recently, cycling coaches were fond of citing the three principles of training: ride, ride, ride. Now we know better. Piling on the mileage—often junk mileage—is rarely the solution. Going faster rather than longer will likely make you a better rider, though this can be a trap too. I ride with a colleague who starts hammering the moment he leaves the driveway and doesn't stop until his house is in sight. He's a strong rider but doesn't get better because he rides the same way all the time. And he hates to rest, another common pitfall for exuberant cyclists.

My friend and many like him are using an old training diary like the Italian cycling manual that warns against sex during peak cycling periods, an admonition that some boxers still adhere to today. Training is not meant to deprive you of the good things in life. Rather, it is meant to *be* a good thing in your life.

You've read stories in this book about people who could hardly walk but could climb aboard the bike and turn the pedals. Some could literally do no more than that. This is, of course, the wonder of cycling. The bike carries your weight, and the gearing lets you improve your performance incrementally. Your joints are not damaged. Your mobility is out in front of you.

The ease with which one can mount a bike and pedal doesn't mean you should start a training program willy-nilly. If you are under a doctor's care or have an ailment, please consult with him or her before starting a cycling program. That said, be wary of some advice you get from the medical community. My family doctor who has been seeing me for twenty-five years is still not an advocate of my exercise regimen. We joke about it. Use your good judgment. I've encountered too many success stories to believe there is any downside to cycling.

Ultimately, even with the help of a compassionate doctor, I believe your fitness and health rest squarely in your hands. A strenuous cycling program will require you to be conscious of your heart rate, resting pulse, recovery time, weight, fat-to-lean body mass, cholesterol, diet, nutrition, mental state, stress levels, and the like, a scrutiny that doctors should applaud. You can indeed monitor your health. For proof of this, listen to Ralphe Gagnon of Hemet, California, who twenty years ago weighed 205 pounds (he's 5′ 8″), smoked cigars, ate badly, led a stressful life, and was told by his cardiologist that a heart attack or stroke was inevitable. After cycling his way back to health, Gagnon is 143 pounds. His blood pressure is 120/70. Pulse rate: 54–60 bpm. According to his doctor, his tests and exams are textbook data.

My point is that you are the author of the fitness textbook. Of course we all want the assurance of a doctor from time to time but the data the physician generates on us is not magical; it reflects our commitment to fitness and health, which goes far beyond cycling. The bike is the vehicle to health but the brain plays a role too. Gagnon lost 60 pounds by cycling 300 miles a month but also by keeping his fat intake to 15 percent of his daily caloric intake. Become a better cyclist and you'll become more conscious of other parts of your life. You'll take charge of your life. Visits to the doctor will likely be less frequent but more rewarding. You don't have to wait for the nurse to tell you your blood pressure, resting pulse, and weight. That information will be in your training diary, where it will do the most good.

Perry Suzanne Templeton of Thibodaux, Louisiana, lost her right foot at the ankle fifteen years ago in a horse accident. Though her orthopedist "saved" the foot "with great difficulty," she couldn't walk normally and sometimes couldn't walk at all. Eight years ago she was given an old heavy ten-speed and she acknowledges making all the typical mistakes: big gears, low cadence, poor bike fit. Nonetheless she rode every day. Then, she reports, a "miraculous thing happened— that sweaty, rambunctious kid in me was reborn. I bought a good mountain bike and a road bike. I ate better, slept great, and embraced a more positive outlook on everything in general.

"I have my good days and horrible days but the more I ride, the better off I am. I rode my first century last year. Cycling makes me equal, whole, and without limitations. It is a forgiving endeavor and soothes my soul. Cycling restored my health, salvaged my sanity, and most importantly reunited me with that sweaty, happy, rambunctious kid."

So to say that anyone can cycle, that cycling meets us at our level of needs, that a person can cycle when she can't walk are not hyperbole. They are truths written large in the pain, will, and motivation of thousands of people I've met and corresponded with. I do not exaggerate when I say that, for many, cycling is a true salvation.

You now know that cycling is an easy sport to start because it is a soft exercise and forgiving. When you are equipped with the right bike and skills, your training becomes that much easier, though given the joy people feel in the sport, play might be a better word. Few people can ignore the child within when they are on a bike.

Anyone who can get on a bike and has the motivation can eventually get it right. I'd like to save you that time. I'd like your passage to cycling to be not just pain-free but joyous. But even joy takes some planning. The heart of a training schedule is time in the saddle. First some tips to ensure that is where you are parked.

I can talk all I want about duration, frequency, and intensity of exercise, the three-horned toad of a training program, but first of all you have to find the time, which is everyone's bane. Mine too. I'm often out at 4:30 A.M. on a Sunday morning so I can be back from a long ride about the same time my daughter Deirdre wakes up. Other times during the week I have to snatch and grab hours. Here are some of my tricks to get my mileage in.

1. Commuting. Without the miles I get from commuting to work, my cycling fitness would suffer greatly. I have a perfect 17-mile commute one way through lightly trafficked roads. I realize most of you might have stiffer challenges. But you could try to commute at least a few times a week. Though these might not be high-quality miles, given the stopping and starting in traffic, they are miles. You can throw in occasional interval spurts between telephone poles to get your pulse up.

2. Goals. Without goals, you'll be meandering all over the road. Decide early on whether you want to do a century or metric century ride on the road or an equivalent off-road distance and plan for it. September and October are the traditional times for centuries though you can find them in most areas as early as June. Look for off-road tours or mountain bike citizen races in your neighborhood but do something. I remember appearing on CNN and announcing before I had really decided that I was planning to ride Land's End to John o'

Groat's. After it was on the air, there was no backing down. Do tell your friends. The pressure will do you good.

3. Lunch Rides. If you can work out the logistics, this is a great way to get in high-intensity miles. Within minutes of my office is a steep hill that I frequently ride during lunch (when I'm not on the trails). Your neighborhood has a spot to challenge you. Find it.

4. Rest. Of course, resting won't put miles on your bike but will likely bring you back refreshed for a longer training ride the next day. I've known countless people who were forced to take off long stretches owing to injuries or personal responsibilities and all have come back stronger.

5. Inside Ride. There is an assortment of bikes on the market that you can ride inside. You can even adapt your road bike, and I'll be talking about these options later. Just keep in mind that though indoor riding is not as thrilling as outside, with care you can still get a brisk workout.

6. Quality. I know professional road cyclists who used to ride 800–1,000 miles a week though most now acknowledge that was not quality mileage. Consequently, the trend for all cyclists is for fewer but better miles. As I'll discuss in Chapter 8, using a heart rate monitor is one way to get the most out of even a thirty-minute ride. A monitor helps you keep most of the workout in the training target zone, which is 60–85 percent of your maximum heart rate.

7. Beater Bike. I have an old 35-pound Fuji with fenders, mudguards, rear rack, and lights to use in inclement weather. When I won't take out my Trek 5500, I will venture out with my Fuji, which has served me for almost ten years. I also have a Raleigh mountain bike I use for the same purpose. So get a beater bike for bad weather. You'll get in the mileage and your bike won't know the difference. By the way, a lot of cyclists use their sturdy mountain bike too in the off-season and off-weather.

8. Halfway. Try cycling to a destination and meeting your family there. It really works. I've saved more family hassles doing this over the years. Often it means getting up early and out hours before the rest of the family but you can still have most of the day with them.

9. Tow Truck. If you have young children, consider buying a trailer so you can tow them behind you while cycling. Cannondale and Burley have fine models on the market. I used a Cannondale Bugger with both my son and daughter. But be careful: it can become addictive. I was still lugging Declan around when he was eight and my daughter Deirdre one. But it's a great workout and a special way to be with your children.

10. Cut Down. If you're cycling 100 miles a week in four days, try doing it in three. You save time and likely become a better cyclist.

Over time you'll discover your own tricks to getting on the bike often, without disrupting the rest of your life. In the process, you'll find shortcuts to better riding, allowing you to take full advantage of time in the saddle. Here are a few I've used successfully over the years.

1. Clockwork. Rather than concentrating on miles, think about minutes when you ride, because the former encourages "junk miles" and burnout. Say to yourself, "I'm going out for an hour," rather than for 20 miles. You'll use the time better and training will be more beneficial.

2. Off-road. Most road riders know that riding a mountain bike off-road will improve bike handling, balance, and upper body strength.

3. Clubs. Join a cycling club. You'll cycle more often and get better in the process. I learn a lot from watching how someone handles a bike.

4. Hills. Ride them at least twice a week. You'll get better, faster.

90

5. Gearing. By now you should have analyzed the bike's gearing to make sure it matches your needs. Don't be reluctant to tape the gear chart on the stem until you know it by heart.

My goal every time I get on a bike is to make the ride a great one. However, how one lives off the bike will have a lot to say about the quality of training. Though some cyclists still boast that "I can eat and drink what I want when I'm cycling," that contention is not borne out by either scientific research or research I've conducted among recreational cyclists.

ALCOHOL

If you drink a lot of alcohol on a Friday night, there's no way you'll have a good ride on Saturday. That's a fact borne out by U.S. Navy research, an outfit that knows something about carousing (I spent four years in the Navy and can vouch for the quality of the research). A Russian friend told me a story about a Russian athlete who stayed up all night drinking vodka before an Olympic final, then turned in her best time in the 10,000-meter run. I'm sure the story is apocryphal. More reliable research indicates that alcohol disturbs the level of iron and trace minerals, thus impairing performance.

As most people know, alcohol dehydrates you. To metabolize one ounce of alcohol, you need to drink eight ounces of water. *Bicycling* magazine surveyed and followed for a season a group of fast recreational riders and all reported bad rides after imbibing the night before.

Marijuana users are no better off, according to a Canadian study, with perception, muscle strength, and balance impaired. Cocaine stimulates the central nervous system, masking the onset of fatigue and encouraging harder training than would be warranted.

This is no lecture. I've had bad rides too and I know this research is true. If you want to be a good rider, eliminate or go easy on the bad stuff. I've found two beers is my limit the night before a ride, but I always ride better without.

SLEEP

Every athlete has a theory about sleep. One I believed for years is that it's important to get a good night's sleep two nights before a big event. However, there's no medical evidence to support it. The fact is strength, aerobic ability, and heart rate change very little even after 50–60 hours of sleep deprivation. Cyclists who participate in the Race Across America (RAAM) have long known that sleep deprivation primarily has psychological effects. In that spirit, the crew of John Marino, who in 1978 set a transcontinental record of a little over 13 days, told him he was sleeping 6 hours a night though he was really sleeping 2. He woke up from these naps refreshed, ready to go. This story is not unusual. I was there for part of the ride and saw the effects.

Most of you won't be racing the clock across country so there's no need to play that game. Research has shown that a regular nap can make up for lost sleep. And to improve the quality of your sleep, ride in the morning rather than at night. Eschew sleeping pills because they deprive you of the deep dream sleep so essential to psychological well-being. Taking a warm bath before bedtime helps. Most of all take heart: Genetics largely determines your sleep requirements. So, don't lose any sleep over lost sleep.

By the time they reach adulthood, though, most people know whether they are morning or night people. And the older you are, the less sleep you need. Research has shown that night people ride better in the evenings and their best cycling season is midsummer. If you're a morning person, you'll have your best rides early, an advantage since that's when most rides start.

CAFFEINE

Caffeine is a stimulant that helps release fatty acids into the bloodstream, thus sparing the carbohydrate store, your most efficient fuel. Few cyclists have not experienced the lift caffeine gives after a long ride. The downside is increased urination, insomnia, and nervousness, depending on how you handle the stimulant. More recent research indicates that caffeine is unnecessary if you are on a high carbohydrate, low-fat diet. For those who want the real caffeine kick, researchers suggest you abstain for four days and then start again. Others suggest the best time for caffeine is 2–3 hours before riding. That's 3–4 cups of coffee, mind you, so be prepared to stop a few times. But in moderation, caffeine can give your ride a boost.

HEALTH

If you're healthy, you'll ride better. If you have a cold, it's best to stay off the bike. Flu viruses can travel to muscles, causing microscopic damage and fatigue. But it's hard to do. I have the flu as I write this and will stop in a few hours to ride my exercise bike easily. If you're going to ride while you're ill, take it gently. Viruses can sap your strength by as much as 15 percent and impair aerobic metabolism.

Fatigue can also be a culprit, taking the joy out of a ride. We know that unstressed athletes have greater aerobic capacity, and exercise is one of the best ways to reduce stress. However, riding when fatigued can increase your stress level. Better to take the day off. Your goal is to be relaxed both on and off the bike. After all, that's one reason you exercise.

Women find that menstruation increases stress levels, and while it does not impair aerobic capacity, it increases their chances for an unsatisfactory ride. So, if you cycle, don't look for a peak performance ride. Otherwise, there are few hindrances to women engaging in hard rides. Many women have found they can cycle well into the third trimester of pregnancy because the bike is literally carrying the weight.

THE ELEMENTS

The weather, terrain, and elements can have as much to do with the quality of the ride as what you eat or drink the night before. My research has shown that, not surprisingly, rides that were rated highly often occurred on sunny days, and those rated poor were in rain or under cloudy skies. Headwinds definitely contribute to a poor ride, though respondents prefer hills over flat courses, a preference I roundly support—I can't stand being stranded on the flatlands. Distance was a factor. Cyclists riding 30 miles tended to enjoy the ride more than those who rode farther. And you're more likely to enjoy the ride when you're with someone of equal ability or a club. Cycling with someone you can't keep up with is definitely demoralizing and a quick way to kill the pleasure. Pick a riding companion of equal ability or one that will push you a little but not to the point of frustration and anger. Yes, I've been there.

Pick the course carefully. You'll enjoy the ride more if you share the road with fewer cars.

And by all means plan. Poor rides tend to be those planned in less than an hour, hardly enough time to prepare. If you are likely to ride on short notice, at least have your bike ready, waiting by the door. Jumping on the bike and riding 50–60 miles is usually an invitation for trouble.

Research indicates that those who leave the watch at home have more enjoyable rides. When you have time to spare and don't have to rush back to take the kids to soccer, try it.

After all my years in the sport, I'm still surprised that while skiing, golf, and tennis have hundreds of camps and instructional schools, cycling, a far more technically demanding sport, has so few. While that situation is changing for the better, most of us are destined to be our own coach, trainer, and fitness expert. To help you gain a broader perspective on training, let me share some ideas I've picked up from coaches, trainers, and Olympians over the years.

OVERALL FITNESS

There's a reason Olympic cyclists at the Colorado Training Camp do more than ride road and mountain bikes. They do weight training, and they play soccer and basketball in the off-season. By the time they are ready to get on their bikes seriously, they have an athletic base to build on. Most cyclists have poor overall fitness, lacking upper body and abdominal strength, and reflexes for superior bike handling. I encourage you to participate in other activities during the season as well. I run, play some soccer, use the stair climber, lift free weights, and do a lot of sit-ups. When I'm conscientious, I notice the difference in my bike handling and on-bike strength.

Road racers are becoming much more enamored of the mountain bike because it forces muscles to work at different angles as your center of gravity changes.

TRAINING ZONES

This option is recommended by coaches for those who choose not to use a heart rate monitor. Mike Deveka, who used to coach Greg LeMond's team, recommends different levels of effort within five training zones. The first zone is one of easy riding. The second is a rate you can maintain for 3–4 hours without getting out of breath. The third is a cycling level you can keep up for 30–60 minutes. The fourth is similar to an interval you can hold for 5 minutes, and the fifth is a hard sprint that lasts no more than 30 seconds. With practice, the Zone Theory will make sense. You might exercise in Zone 1 the day after a hard ride. Zone 2 might be your weekend endurance ride. Zone 3 requires a stiff training pace. Zones 4 and 5 give you the zip.

Please remember that these training zones are similar to the "intensity levels" discussed in Chapter 9.

STRENGTH AND SPEED

Most cyclists don't improve because they don't vary their training sufficiently. For variety, pick a hill that's between 1 and 2 miles and climb it while seated pedaling at 60 rpm. A week later ride the same hill in the next hardest gear at the same cadence. If you fall below 60 rpm, downshift. The next week, use the same drill. You can use this tactic, particularly in the early season, on both the road and the single track to build strength.

For speed on the road, though the carryover to mountain biking should be obvious, do speed workouts consisting of three 200- to 500-meter sprints at 85 percent of capacity after a warm-up. Spin easier between efforts to recover. As your training improves, increase the number of sprints and the intensity. Well into the season some cyclists like to do "sprint pyramids" on safe, traffic-free roads where equally spaced telephone poles are often available as markers. The drill is simple. After a warm-up, sprint at 80 percent of maximum for one section, spin to recover for three; sprint one, recover two, sprint one, recover one; sprint one, recover two, sprint one and recover for three. Sprint one and cool down. Weekly sprint sessions will put snap in your legs and improve your speed. And you don't even need a coach.

CYCLE TRAINING

Most of us follow the clock, training in weekly cycles, easy in the beginning, hard at the end. Usually this regimen means rest on Monday, speed work on Wednesday, and long rides on Sunday. There's nothing wrong with that except that some coaches think it's not the best and surest route to fitness. Instead of thinking of a week's training program, you might want to think of training in 5-week cycles, especially if you want to race. Let's say you've come off a series of hard rides or a race. Use Week 1 to rest and recover, cycling at about 50 percent of your maximum. Week 2 is for rebuilding. Distance and intensity at 75 percent of maximum. Weeks 3 and 4 you prepare for your event. If you're preparing for a century, do one long ride each week. One hundred miles is ideal but there's nothing wrong with a stiff 50- to 75-mile ride. If your goal is to participate in a fast club ride, concentrate on interval training and speed work. And Week 5 is for tapering, riding at 70 percent of maximum intensity. You should feel as if you are holding back. Coaches say it's like holding the reins of a horse who has been in the barn too long.

Some of this advice from veteran coaches will apply at different stages of your progress. Consult the advice again when you tend to get stale. Within all this information, you'll find a strategy that works for you. If you ride predominantly off-road, you'll likely ride longer, perhaps harder, but record fewer miles than on the road. Don't worry about it. Mountain biking often provides more overall fitness than road riding, especially at altitude. Modify any program that doesn't meet your needs. If something doesn't work for you, ignore it. Your best guide is your common sense and how you feel. The more confident you become, the more issue you'll take with the experts, including me.

Whatever bike you ride, whatever cycling objective you hold, and whatever long-term plan you have for your health and fitness, you must build a foundation of miles on the bike. Time in the saddle is where fitness begins. Again, cycling meets you at your level of need. If you're reasonably fit, are presently engaged in other strenuous aerobic activities, there is probably no reason you can't get on a bike and ride 10 miles. As always, your fitness and health should be a determining factor. Don't do anything stupid. If you are significantly overweight, have heart problems and the like, you should check with a doctor. That's my obligatory statement. On the other hand, don't baby yourself. The bike is easy, gentle exercise. You control the speed and, through the gears, the workload. The secret is brisk pedaling in low gears, precisely the way racers have trained for decades because it conditions muscles, heart, lungs, and buttocks.

For example, if you are coming off a winter layoff or have been doing light aerobic work, you'll want to begin your spring thing riding four or five days a week, say for the first six weeks. Monday, Wednesday, and Friday would be off days with one being optional. Pick a mileage level you're comfortable with and start there the first week. For example, if you plan to ride 50 miles during Week 1, try to ride 10 percent more Week 2. By the end of your Week 6 plateau, you'll be close to 80 miles. Modify the mileage if you plan to do all your riding off-road. The principle is the same: The first six weeks should consist of easy pedaling in low gears, say 60 inches or 42×18T. Try to avoid hills, but if you must climb, easy does it. Don't be tempted to take a flyer with your friends or ride a tough single track before you are ready. A bright spring day is often the only stimulant needed to turn a ride into a race. Resist the temptation.

97

After Week 6 you should add another riding day to your menu and increase the intensity a bit. Continue to increase your mileage by 10 percent a week so that you'll be at 120 miles a week by Week 10. You have more than doubled your mileage in eight weeks. Now you should specialize the training a little more.

MONDAY. If you are following the Monday–Sunday sequence, this is your rest day. New cyclists often overtrain. Don't.

TUESDAY. A 20-mile ride with 3–4 thirty-second sprints thrown in mid-ride. Concentrate on pedal cadence.

WEDNESDAY. An easy 15-mile ride in low gears.

THURSDAY. A 20–25-mile ride with hills or longer intervals. Find two or three long hills you can climb at a steady cadence. Or find a stretch where you can time-trial for 2 five–minute periods in a large gear at 80 rpm.

FRIDAY. Off or a short, easy ride of 10 miles.

SATURDAY. A long, steady endurance ride of 35 miles. Try to stay in low gears and avoid too many hills. You'll likely be out for at least two hours, so don't forget to take some fruit or an energy bar.

SUNDAY. A 20-mile ride, ideally with friends, so you can practice riding in a paceline or a pack, or sprinting between various road markers. Go 10–15 miles if you are riding off-road.

Again, if you are mixing road and off-road miles, adjust the mileage accordingly. You'll get a harder workout for fewer miles on the mountain than on the road. Mountain biking requires greater focus and intensity and that is why mountain bike racers often spend 50 percent of their time on the road, just exchanging the knobby tires for slick ones.

Wherever you cycle or whatever you ride, the principles are the same. Go easy in the early season, concentrating on spinning in low gears. Get the base mileage. Add some speciality training as you develop a foundation. Stay with the 10 percent rule.

After Week 10, you're ready for a long ride such as a century or a multiple-day tour. If you plan to do a mountain bike tour or enter a citizen's race, you will want to hone the skills discussed in the last chapter as you build your mileage base. Skill building is a daily activity for all cyclists. There's always something new to learn.

Famed mountain bike coach Skip Hamilton reminds us of the limits of rigid training programs. "Don't blindly copy the top riders' training. Durango locals like to ride John Tomac's wheel out to Mesa Verde, but two weeks later, they're fried. We love to emulate our heroes, and we can base our training on the same principles. We just can't do as much or go as fast.

"Most riders go too easy on their hard days and too hard on their easy days. We find it difficult to go slowly, but easy days need to be guilt-producing slow. Use your heart rate monitor to slow you. Overdress so it's uncomfortable to go fast or ride with someone much slower than you are."

Good advice. The more you know about yourself and the more carefully you monitor your overall fitness and health, the less likely you will be to slavishly follow advice from any source, including this book, which is meant to empower, not enslave, you.

As a coda to this chapter, let me add a few specific training programs from a range of recreational riders so you have an idea what people in our shoes are doing. I'm inspired by the Olympians but more likely to emulate specific examples of my peers, who work a full week and still manage to ride 5,000 miles a year.

JAMES C. McCULLAGH

Case Study 1

Patrick King of Highland, Vermont, has been cycling seriously
for the last six years and has ridden as much as 7,000 miles
annually. He's completed ten centuries and ridden 158 miles in
a day. He's a stickler for keeping a log, knowing exactly what
level of training he's been doing for the last six years. He even
keeps a record of his climbs with an Avocet 50 Cyclometer. He
rides through the winter except when the roads are icy. He's
using a modified three-week training program, leading up to
long rides at the end cycle. What follows is a typical June
schedule he was shooting for. By the way, he doesn't ride on
Sunday so is obliged to increase his miles during the week.
Keep in mind this assumes a significant foundation of miles.

	S	M	T	W	T	F	S
Week 1	R	R	R	25	R	R	100
Week 2	R	30	60	90	30	30	150
Week 3	R	50	60	150	30	30	200
Week 4	R	R	R	30	50	200	200

I haven't heard whether this program was successful, but given
King's past accomplishments, I have no reason to doubt him.
The point is not his high mileage, but the alternate rest and
training days. He begins the training cycle with a lot of rest and
tapers at the end with three rest days before his final long ride.

Study the principle, not the content. You can put any mileage
on the chart. King commutes to work, a 60-mile round trip, and
can pile on the mileage. This schedule reflects contemporary
thinking that suggests you might be better off looking at your
training schedule in chunks of weeks and months, rather than
days. This encourages a long view and forces rest days, which
are as important as those on the bike.

If you're organized, like to keep records, hold a long view of

100

training, and feel this kind of cycle would suit you, have a go. But base your mileage on your goals and your cycling habits. Remember King is doing all his cycling on a road bike. The mileage would look quite different if he included some mountain bike training.

The basis of this program is physiologically sound as it encourages rest and schedules the long rides in cycles the body seems to readily accept. Coaches who have used this method or a modified version report fewer injuries among their athletes, so it's definitely worth experimenting with.

Case Study 2

Nicholas Cheek of Lincolnton, North Carolina, has been cycling nine years, averaging 2,000 miles annually. He rides at least six centuries a year and has ridden 120 miles in a day. His primary bike is a tandem. His Kestrel 200 SCi is displayed in his theological library. He describes his training program:

"Although 80 to 85 percent of my cycling is on a Santana tandem, we still ride a road bike. Our peak cycling season begins in April and continues through October. We do not use a time schedule on a training ride. We base our warm-ups, training performance, and cool down upon miles ridden. I am blessed with two stokers, my wife and daughter, which also creates two different methods of training. Warm-up consists of 3–6 miles. Performance consists of 1–15 miles at 90 to 100 rpm. Here we include sprints for 30 seconds, resting for 90 seconds, and repeat 5 times. At this point we return to 90 to 100 rpm for 3–5 miles and repeat at least twice on a 25- to 40-mile ride. When riding a tandem, hill climbing, gear changes, and momentum into the hill become a training specialty for any team."

There is a gentleness and a reality to this training schedule. Nicholas Cheek and his wife put their relationship at the center of the training regimen but at the same time have an enviable strategy to improve their performance. Minister Cheek, God forbid, is not about to let some ordinary road rider pass him, particularly on the downhills.

Case Study 3

Chris Etue of St. Marys, Ontario, has been cycling seriously for ten years. She rides on average 3,000 miles a year, has completed at least two centuries, and has ridden as far as 110 miles in a day. She plays ice hockey three times a week and says she has no rigid training program.

She rides 3–4 times a week, 18–30 miles each time (15–18 miles on the mountain bike). These are mostly solitary training rides at 60–90 percent of maximum heart rate (she uses a heart rate monitor). Once or twice a week she does hard interval training. The remaining rides are recovery or for pleasure. She competes in a duathlon once a month from May to October.

Her mountain bike riding is mainly on gravel roads, often as a recovery ride, and also as a preparation for her one off-road race a year.

Her training is a mixture of fartlek and some intervals. She does group rides and some loaded touring with her family.

I find this training program very balanced, social, and regenerative. She is not interested in the high mileage but in a balanced life. Apparently it works. She admits to having more energy at 40-something than she had at 20. My nonscientific research indicates that women are more social than men and will likely build a training schedule around social activities.

Case Study 4

Michael Tice has cycled for four years, averaging more than 6,000 miles annually. He rides a road and a mountain bike and acknowledges no off-season. Since beginning his cycling program, his weight and blood pressure have dropped. He rides for the peace, for "sorting out the garbage," for the romance. His program:

"I try to ride no more than five days a week and never much more than that. I always do an easy 25–50 miles on Monday to recover from racing or a long (75-mile) club ride on the weekend. Tuesday is sprints and intervals. Wednesday is a very hard, fast, hilly club ride of at least 50 minutes. Thursday can be a rest day or a 30–50-miler but real easy and most often with a friend. We leave the stopwatch at home and have the HRM turned off on this one. Friday is a moderate workout if I'm racing Sunday or I'll ride my mountain bike on trails with my son. Then do a half an hour of sprints or hill climbs. If it's a Saturday race, I'll skip the sweat work and just play Dad. Saturday we race or do a long ride with some jumps. I've learned to be flexible in my training. I ride my MB-2 on the road from November to April, which really seems to keep me strong, and riding in the snow and ice does wonders for your bike-handling skills and reflexes. I also ride the MB-2 for a break sometimes and race off-road when the road season winds down in September. I try to keep a base of 200 miles a week during the season."

Apparently Tice doesn't slow down much in the off-season either, keeping his mileage fairly consistent. But there is plenty of balance to his program. He uses the mountain bike for recovery and skill building. And he keeps his training in perspective.

Case Study 5

John Boone of Machias, Maine, rides about a thousand miles a year, evenly split between his road and his mountain bike. His longest ride to date is 50 miles. He uses his road bike for aerobic conditioning and his mountain bike for social rides and to challenge his navigational skills. He carries his bike a lot when exploring the woods, a quest that began when he was in the fourth grade.

During April to June and September and October, he rides his road bike three days a week, 10–15 miles a day. Sometimes on a Sunday morning or a weekend afternoon, he goes on an exploratory mountain bike ride of 5–10 miles. During the summer he rides the mountain bike for general transportation and for group rides.

This modest training program underscores a significant trend in our sport. People are buying road bikes for aerobic conditioning and mountain bikes for exploring. Single-track riding is an essential part of an overall cycling fitness program, perhaps doing more for one's mental health than all the time you put on the road.

Case Study 6

Ed Pavelka, a longtime friend, colleague, and executive editor for *Bicycling* magazine, specializes in long-distance events. He has completed the Paris–Brest–Paris *randonnée* and the 750-mile Boston–Montreal–Boston, and he has ridden across America. Well into his forties, he seems to get better with age. He has averaged more than 11,000 miles for the last nine years, never going more than four days without being on his bike. Some of our readers are thrilled by his exploits; others tell him to get a life. His program:

"During the off-season, from November through February, I ride 4–5 times per week on the road and go mountain biking on weekends. I don't consider this training as much as enjoying being on a bike. There's no pressure to do a certain workout or go a certain distance. I play it by feel or the weather. Most of these rides are 2–3 hours long, and like every outing in Pennsylvania, they include hills. Climbing contributes to fitness even on these easy pleasure rides. There's no more natural way to get and stay fit than to climb a couple of thousand feet each time you ride.

"March begins the mileage buildup needed for the ultramarathon events I love. Since 1991, I've ridden the International Randonneurs' brevet series each season. These events progress in distance from 125 to 375 miles. Training during this period averages 400–500 miles a week, including back-to-back centuries on weekends. These are steady rides in my aerobic heart rate zone, with care not to exceed the anaerobic threshold on climbs.

"In September and October, I still ride a lot even if there are no events. This is my favorite time of year, so I enjoy it by taking long weekend rides and getting out each evening in the golden autumn sun. In fact, I put on my lighting system so I can ride through the sunset. I also start trail riding on my mountain bike—a great way to see fall colors.

"Throughout the year, I mix in rides on a tandem, going with a friend who also enjoys long distances. On a weekend day we'll often ride 70 to 100 miles. I also have a beater bike with fenders and a rack trunk."

Ed Pavelka's training schedule is a wonder to everyone he works with. Ed has discovered that he excels in ultramarathon events and chases them with a passion. But his program, though consisting of high mileage, is orderly and balanced. His love is the road bike but the mountain bike has opened his eyes. He's stopping to smell the roses, though not for very long. An 11,000-mile year leaves little time for dawdling.

I would not be offended if you considered these training pro-

105

grams a kind of flea market you pick through to find the perfect antique. Or a clothing sale with everything reduced by 50 percent. Charge in, look around, stick the interesting stuff under your arm, and try it on for size. There is a training program for every cyclist, every whim, desire, need, circumstance, and dream. Most of us live in a world restricted by time and responsibilities and make the best of our lot. But as you can see, the married with children can still put in impressive miles without fear of abandoning the children. I have regularly put in 6,000–7,000-mile years while conscientiously raising a son and a daughter.

In cycling, as in life, the end is always the beginning.

Case Study 7

Jim Litterio of Fitchburg, Massachusetts, weighed in at 310 pounds on the morning of his thirtieth birthday. He smoked two packs of cigarettes a day and his cholesterol levels were through the roof. He was laid off.

Something moved Jim to buy a $90 department store bike, and with the help of a healthy diet, he managed to lose 110 pounds. Now, he feels great, has a better bike, and hasn't smoked in two years. He looked so good the local sheriff's department hired him. All this for $90.

Once again: Cycling meets you at your level of need and helps you fly.

In subsequent chapters we'll meet other cyclists who train as if their lives depend on it.

I'll conclude with a few more training programs of editors of *Bicycling* and *Mountain Bike* magazines.

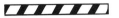

TRAINING PROGRAM 1: FAMILY MAN

This is the training schedule of Joe Kita, until recently executive editor of *Bicycling* magazine. He's a solid fitness cyclist and a family man. His schedule includes both.

January and February

My focus is on strength and power building interspersed with different aerobic activities.

Weight training: 30–40 minutes every other day with a variety of exercises for upper and lower body. High repetitions with light-to-moderate weight are stressed because I'm not out to build bulk.

Aerobic: On rest days from lifting, I'll run, skate, or mountain-bike.

March and April

My focus will gradually shift to road riding and building aerobic endurance.

Road riding: 50–100 miles a week (depending on weather) garnered through commutes and weekend rides. Mostly low-gear, easy spinning work to get cycling muscles back into shape.

Weight training: 30 minutes twice weekly.

May through September

This is peak road-riding season, and I'll do little else.

Road riding: 100–200+ miles a week. Weekends are for long endurance rides or faster group rides/events. Weekdays are for commutes (40 miles round trip, 2–3 times weekly) with interval work interspersed. At least one day a week will be a leisurely family ride, either with my wife on our tandem, my son or daughter on our tandem, or pulling my daughter in a buggy. We'll also do a lot of touring. Easy rides and rest become more important at this time of year because of the intensity of most rides and the pure volume of hours on the bike. Normally, I'll take one day off per week.

October through December

Focus is on enjoying the fitness built during the summer. Centuries, tours, commuting—in all, it's a gradual taper back off the peak and into the winter training schedule. Emphasis is on fun, not preparation.

Road riding: 75–150 miles a week. Most mileage comes through commutes and weekend group or family rides.

Weight training: Twice weekly workouts with gradually building weight as this period progresses.

Mountain biking: This gradually replaces road riding as days shorten and weather gets colder.

Skating and running also start to be done more often for diversions.

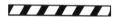

TRAINING PROGRAM 2: HARD CHARGER

This is from Geoff Drake, *Bicycling* editor. He averages about 9,000 miles a year. His racing is almost entirely off-road. He trains with weights and runs year-round.

Monday: Easy run. Lift weights.

Tuesday: Hard ride with heart rate monitor (intervals).

Wednesday: Steady aerobic ride.

Thursday: Hard ride with heart rate monitor (intervals).

Friday: Easy run. Lift weights.

Saturday: Steady aerobic ride.

Sunday: Hard group ride or race.

I ride to work every day. If I go straight in, it's 6 miles each way. To achieve a longer ride, I'll lengthen this in one direction or the other.

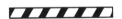

TRAINING PROGRAM 3: TABLE TENNIS PLAYER

This is Jim Langley's schedule. He is a West Coast editor for *Bicycling*, and he rides every day. His training emphasizes being ready to peak in 6 weeks.

Monday: Abdominal routine to prepare my lower back for cycling: hanging from a chin-up bar, 2 sets of 10 "knee-ups" (lifting knees to chest and holding for 1 second, then repeat). In addition, I do:

- 25 slow abdominal curls
- 20 fast abdominal curls
- 25 leg lifts
- 10 push-ups

One-hour easy ride, spinning, enjoying the scenery.

Tuesday: 20-minute run; 1.5-hour off-road ride with climbing; 20 minutes stretching; 2 hours of competition table tennis.

Wednesday: Abdominal routine; 2-hour ride steady (about 17 mph).

Thursday: 20- to 30-minute run; 1-hour ride easy; 20 minutes stretching; 2 hours of competition table tennis.

Friday: Abdominal routing; 1.5-hour ride off-road (fartlek).

Saturday: 3-hour group road ride (race pace); 20-minute jog.

Sunday: 2-hour off-road group ride (fun ride).

TRAINING PROGRAM 4: CRAZY MUSICIAN

Captain Dondo, *Mountain Bike* editor, says:

"I don't train anymore. I've decided that such manic behavior leads me to poor mental and physical health. I do, however, still exercise on a regular basis. Regular exercise leads me to good mental and physical health. I used to train like a maniac for bike racing, but now that I've begun to mature, I find more of my time devoted to other pursuits— my marriage, upkeep of my home, playing guitar, reading philosophy, watching good movies, visiting friends and family, furthering my career, playing with my dog, and meditating. Keeping fit with cycling alone takes more time than I can afford in my new schedule, so my riding is augmented with such low-time/high-quality activities as weight lifting, cross-country skiing, and running."

Winter

Monday A.M.: 1 hour weight lifting—chest, shoulders, triceps, abs—six exercises, 4–5 sets each, 6–15 reps (300–1,000 reps total abs).
    Lunchtime: 40-minute jog—comfortable pace.
Tuesday A.M.: 1 hour weight lifting—legs, lower back, upper back, biceps, abs—8 exercises, 3–5 sets each, 6–15 reps (300 reps abs).
    Lunchtime: 30-minute cross-country ski—comfortable pace.
Wednesday A.M.: 20 minutes windtrainer—easy spin.
Thursday A.M.: Same as Monday.
Friday A.M.: Same as Tuesday.
Saturday or Sunday: 2-hour hike, mountain bike ride, or X-C ski.
The other weekend day: 30 minutes windtrainer ride or jog.

Summer

Monday A.M.: 40-minute road ride.
    Lunchtime: 1 hour weight lifting—full body, 12 exercises, 2 sets each, 12–15 reps.
Tuesday lunchtime: 1- to 1½-hour mountain bike ride. The topography enforces a high level of energy output.
Wednesday A.M.: 30-minute jog.
    Lunchtime: Easy 1-hour road or mountain bike ride.
Thursday A.M.: Weight lifting—same as Monday.
    P.M.: Thursday night ride, or fairly hard mountain bike ride.
Friday: Lunchtime mountain bike or road ride, easy, with a lunch stop.
Saturday or Sunday: 2–6-hour road or mountain bike epic (if I'm lucky).
The other weekend day: 30-minute jog, tennis, or other outdoor recreation.

EPIPHANIES

Every once in a while life shocks us with an epiphany. For Alan Klein of Philadelphia, the epiphany came on his fiftieth birthday, when, out of breath and weighing 238 pounds, he visited his doctor, who said, in so many words, "Change your life or die." Klein did change, joining Weight Watchers and buying a Raleigh mountain bike. He lost 50 pounds and purchased a Cannondale road bike which suited his distance riding ambitions. So he pushed himself and rode farther.

Another epiphany. He had a heart attack while riding with his wife, which would have been much more severe if he had not lost weight and ridden his bike. He underwent quadruple bypass surgery, recovered, and resumed his love affair with the bike. He discovered he had an appetite for long, multiday tours so he purchased a Cannondale ST 1000 touring bike, a little longer than a road bike, which allowed him to carry a pack. He hasn't stopped since, riding in the Glacier National Park in Montana and Waterton Lakes National Park in Alberta, Canada.

As a child, William Moore of Pleasant Hill, California, dreamed of being a Six Day racer and actually became good enough to race on the velodrome on Treasure Island, San Francisco, in 1939 prior to the race won by Killan and Vopel, darlings of Hitler, who declared a holiday in Germany right before he invaded Poland. The war killed the Six Day circuit and Moore's dreams. He didn't ride a bike again until he'd had 60 percent of his lung removed and suffered a heart attack. He made an oath that one day he would ride 21 miles. He sold his sailboat and still wonders how he got through his first 5-mile ride. He did and has averaged about 2,500 miles for the last twenty years.

When illness or injury strikes, we often come to the startling conclusion that our body is the engine that drives us. The television commercial for a fitness club that laments that people are more careful about what they put into their cars than their bodies is unfortunately true. Not long ago I was in a taxi on my way to the Atlanta airport when I felt something was not right—with the car. Small signs at first, such as what sounded like incomplete combustion in the carburetor. I could see the engine was running hot and steam was pouring from the engine before the light came on. Then the car lost oil pressure, conked out, and I had to walk the rest of the way to the airport.

I suspect the taxi just needed a tune-up and maybe a new oil pump. The driver was probably on his way before I got off the ground. The taxi driver ignored the signs of distress, despite my questions, until the car stopped abruptly in a metallic shudder. Sadly, we do the same thing all too often and wait for the mechanic to arrive in the tow truck and announce that we are overweight, with high blood pressure and high cholesterol and all the usual risks of mortality. The ability to endlessly tantalize our immortality is a curious trait of human nature. I once spoke to a U.S. Naval official about preparing health pamphlets for sailors at sea. He laughed and said I'd have to wait until they were in their forties because it is only then that mortality strikes. Yes, I remember, having spent four years at sea in the Pacific, relentlessly daring all the gods. But I still fantasize about living forever, though friends and family continue to die at an altogether regular pace. Change is hard and often comes at a cost we're unwilling to pay. A good friend of mine just got divorced because the wife he loved very much was serving him too much rich food and drink. No kidding. Her idea of a future was to grow fat together into old age and refused to adjust her cooking or alcohol consumption. Not surprisingly, my friend's epiphany came as he walked away from the newly dug grave of his sister.

Imagine a firefighter weighing 250 pounds who had difficulty going up and down stairs without getting winded. Meet Dennis Symons, Jr., of Robbinsville, New Jersey, who decided that, as a career firefighter, he was in unacceptable condition. He did not wait for the tow truck to pull up to his door. He bought a Diamond Back mountain bike, rode four miles, and thought he was going to die. Within a year he had lost 50 pounds, primarily through cycling. Hooked, he purchased a Cannondale R-1000, which cost him $2,000, about the same amount he had spent on useless diet programs. To date, he has lost 75 pounds and has become a legitimate mountain bike racer. His friends consider him a nut but he is alive and well.

I love to hear from people who begin at the very beginning by cycling one mile. Such a story belongs to Mark Blaisdell of East Kingston, New Hampshire, who, weak and concerned, visited his doctor and was told he had high blood pressure, a blood sugar level of 400 (normal range is 80–120), and a cholesterol level of 295. Determined to do something about it, he purchased a blood glucose monitor and cut out trips to the doughnut shop and fast-food restaurants. He increased his cycling mileage from a dead stop to 2,200 miles in a little over a year. He was able to discontinue his oral blood sugar medication, but his doctor was suspicious of the results and ordered independent tests. Here they are:

	Before	After
Weight	240	196
Blood Sugar	400	70–90
Cholesterol	295	184
Blood Pressure	160/95	135/85
Resting Pulse	90	72

You need to know absolutely nothing about medicine to recognize that Blaisdell is in better shape than he was two years ago. Though he is still taking one blood pressure tablet a day, he has made significant health strides. He took charge of his health, and instead of initiating a regimen of insulin injections, as his doctor recommended, he decided to monitor his blood sugar level and adjust his diet. He got his diabetes under control. One thing leads to another. Lose weight and usually your cholesterol, blood pressure, and resting pulse will come down. This is not black magic.

Blaisdell is an example of an individual who not only is taking charge of his health with a cornerstone built on cycling, but has assumed a role traditionally reserved for doctors in America. However, with the advent of technology and home-monitoring systems, there is no reason that, with proper instruction and oversight, we can't do more to monitor our health. A *Bicycling* magazine reader told me a long time ago, "The only time I visit my family doctor is to show him what great shape I'm in. It's worth the $30." Beyond the hubris, there is a point behind the remarks of my spendthrift friend. There's nothing particularly mysterious about the baselines of health, as recorded above. We'd all be more virtuous if we had a better understanding of lipoproteins and the like, but one doesn't need a medical degree to monitor his or her health. That's a health care plan all of us can live with.

I am a runner and truly love the sport, so I have no intention of comparing it unfavorably with cycling. The two sports are just different. Perhaps the difference is in my often-repeated refrain: Cycling meets us at our level of need. Sadly, not everyone can run, especially those who are heavy or have injuries that intervene. I know of the runner's high and have felt it on occasion. I've also felt it on a bike but what I feel most often is regeneration and the belief that the bike can really help make me over. Cycling contributes to our physical, psychological, and spiritual health in ways not fully understood. When I insist that cycling is for everyone, I don't mean to imply that other activities are not. I simply mean that cycling is an easy sport to start, stay with, and excel at.

This story belongs to Inge Peeters of Oostende, Belgium, who was hit by a car while riding her bike and seriously injured. The list: seven fractures of the spinal column, four broken ribs, fractured right shoulder, concussion, and damaged lungs. No wonder she had a "near death" experience. Confined to bed for months, she had to relearn all the basic motor movements as if she were child. Slowly, she learned to walk again. Two years later she is back on the bike racing. She still is in pain and often feels despair, but the bike is a drug that keeps her focused.

Austin Clark of Pueblo, Colorado, knows something about regeneration. He had routine surgery to help straighten his leg, which in the process became paralyzed. After visits to the usual round of specialists, the pain continued, the leg was still paralyzed, and the muscles started to atrophy. A cyclist, he taped the paralyzed leg to the pedal and started riding again. He couldn't walk or run but could ride with a nonfunctioning leg taped to the pedal.

He rode every day and noticed, with his increased mileage, the pain lessened. But the paralysis continued and the prognosis was not good. Then one night eighteen months after surgery, he felt his little toe move and watched it breathlessly the rest of the night. Gradually the nerve regenerated and he has nearly 100 percent use of his leg to take him on his weekly road and mountain bike rides of 150–250 miles. He said, "Bicycling helped regenerate my injured nerve and soul. It helped me feel whole again. Now I know why they say bicycling is a lifetime sport."

As a writer and editor who has worked in and around the medical field for almost twenty years, I have a good knowledge of the medical literature and constantly learn from it. I'm especially up-to-date on research having to do with cycling, which is marked by its paucity. With a Ph.D. in philosophy, I have a passion for research and am a rabid student of the scientific methods. However, I cannot ignore the anecdotal information that has been pouring across my desk for the last fifteen years. I've seen too many examples of cycling bringing people back to life and have confirmed these examples with the medical community. Because cycling is gentle, flowing, and forgiving, it talks to the body perhaps on a cellular level. That is, at least, my theory. Gaining health and fitness is about time and patience, and the bike is a patient being. Not for a minute am I suggesting the bicycle replace a doctor's care. That would be silly. Ironically, the bicycle often comes in when the doctor's care runs out. But this is not to disparage doctors who must deal with heroic medicine. Cycling seems to intervene very quietly and slowly in a decidedly unheroic manner. As cyclists have told me, the activity allows the body to remember the rudimentary act of pedaling, possibly from an earlier age. Many people have told me that their legs remembered how to cycle before their brains did. But does cycling heal or encourage the body to heal and regenerate itself?

Tom Mueller of Oshkosh, Wisconsin, thinks so. A mountain bike racer, triathlete, and ultradistance runner, he suddenly lost all feeling and balance, and was diagnosed with Guillain-Barré syndrome, a nerve disorder that causes antibodies to eat the sheaves off the nerve endings, causing the entire body to short-circuit. He was left with a slight twitch in his fingers. His breathing went, and he was put on a respirator for nine days. Within a month he was on an exercise bike pushing himself against the advice of the therapist. After his release from the hospital, he got in extra workouts at the local YMCA. Within three months, he was back at work with an eye to a 7-day, 500-mile event. He knows his recovery would not have been as fast and sure without the bicycle.

So does Bernard Greenberg of Highlands Ranch, Colorado, a bike racer who suddenly experienced numbness in his feet and hands. He could hardly walk. Doctors diagnosed multiple sclerosis (MS) and said he would probably never be able to ride his bike again. He was told not to exercise. After a few months of drug therapy, Greenberg started to lift weights and went for an 8-mile ride on a local bike path. He gradually worked up from 20 miles a week to 115. He notes, "I don't know if my recovery and ability to maintain remission from MS are solely the responsibility of my bike and cycling, but I do know that without them I would have been lost and unable to function." And perhaps that's enough.

I mean this chapter as an interlude before we start pushing the big gears again, shedding weight, eating smarter, and riding harder. If cycling did little more than improve one's cardiovascular conditioning, it might not have such appeal. It's because cycling can transform a life and make one whole again that people sing its praises.

GAUGES

I cycle with a friend who is fireplug short with piston legs. He's a strong rider who can do century rides for a week and keep going. He has broken enough chains to keep the Uniglide factory working overtime. He's a good cyclist but doesn't seem to get better, in part because he doesn't want to. He's perfectly happy grinding out the miles.

My friend would be quite at home with cycling groups anywhere in the country because the tendency among enthusiasts is to pile on the miles, and to pay too little attention to the quality. He cycles miles out of his way to avoid climbing a hill, though he takes pleasure roaring past me down the other side.

More than one coach has told me that endurance riding is easy, speed riding is hard. And I've fallen victim to the mileage syndrome, paying more attention to my cyclometer than my heart rate. Mike Walden, the dean of American cycling coaches, has trained more than 300 cyclists who won medals in national and world championship events. Lesson 1 underscores his entire philosophy of coaching: Be your own coach. And he is not being blithe or fanciful. You must learn to coach yourself. What Walden means is that you should keep a detailed log book of your daily rides, thoroughly understand the gearing and how it relates to your particular pedaling ability, monitor your heart rate religiously, and keep a record of your food intake. And while you're at it, consider the three most common mistakes new riders make: underinflating their tires, taking an incorrect position on the bike, and developing an inefficient pedaling stroke using the

117

wrong gears. He's such a stickler on correct pedaling that the coach doesn't even let his riders train in the big chainring. "You must first learn how to pedal quickly, then you can slow it down and develop power," he advises.

If one common syndrome among recreational cyclists is piling on the "junk miles," the other is overtraining, which is essentially not listening to your body. But how *do* you listen to your body? If our sleep is off, our mood sour, our nerves edgy, we know something is wrong but can only guess if and how it's related to our training. On a simpler level, I have spoken of hard and easy days. How is one to know an easy day from a hard day? And how do I know when I should abandon the bike for a couple of days?

One answer is to build an intimate relationship with your heart—that mighty muscle that flexes on your behalf 100,000 times a day and sends more than 4,000 gallons of blood through 60,000 miles of veins, capillaries, and arteries. On average, the heart beats 70 times a minute at rest, adding up to that whopping six-figure number mentioned above. That's for the average person. A world-class cyclist's heart might beat only 40 times a minute at rest, which means it beats much less than the heart of a sedentary person.

Cycling benefits the heart in a number of ways. The heart muscle itself becomes thicker and stronger, output is increased, resting heart rate diminishes, capillaries increase, blood pressure decreases, and aerobic (oxygen-carrying) capacity rises. If you are a new cyclist, you are likely to show a 20 percent gain in aerobic power during the first four months of training, though progress is much slower after that.

The point is this baby should be watched, pampered, encouraged, fed, and measured on a regular basis because, if the eyes are the windows to your soul, the heart is the window to your aerobic conditioning and health. Don't be afraid to look inside. The swampy beats you hear are really the breath of life.

Earlier I mentioned the three pillars of training: frequency, duration, and intensity. Frequency means how often you do something; duration—how long in miles, minutes, or hours; and intensity—often it's anyone's guess. Actually, you do have a built-in monitor to measure training intensity; it's your heart and it knows all. Your heart knows that, in order to get a training effect, it must work at 65 percent of the maximum. That is where real training and conditioning begin. Conversely, the reason most people on bikes don't get any significant aerobic benefit is that they tool along in a low or middle gear never getting their heart rate near this 65 percent level.

So knowing your heart rate through phases of training is fundamental. To find your maximum heart rate, you can get a stress test. A simpler rule of thumb is to subtract your age from 220 and multiply by 0.65 and 0.85 to determine the target heart rate zone. This information is usually available on all health club walls, reminding us that we should "stay between the lines." As you know, you can determine your heart rate by checking the pulse at the neck (carotid artery) or at the wrist. Count the number of beats in 15 seconds and multiply by 4. You've probably seen the nurse in the doctor's office do this often enough.

Better still you can buy for as little as $65 a commercial heart rate monitor, which usually consists of a transmitter strapped to the chest and a receiver for the wrist. The heart rate reading is displayed on the face of the receiver. Many of the cyclists you've met so far in the book have successfully used heart rate monitors to record the quality of their training. So it's easy and within reach of everyone.

More coaches are throwing out the formulas in favor of individualized data, which takes into account individual differences. The above formula is safe, but doesn't take into account various exigencies. For example, what about the 220 minus age rule if your pulse is naturally high? Or conversely, too low? If that's the case, the standard training ranges might be too easy. To counter that, Rory O'Reilly, former Olympic track champion, suggests a maximum heart rate test but only for the well conditioned, not for the faint of heart. Here a doctor's approval is on order. You already have your heart rate monitor. O'Reilly recommends using a stationary trainer and a friend to assist. Aim to reach your maximum in about 15 minutes. Pedal to reach a heart rate of 120–130 bpm, within easy reach of most. Your cadence is 80–90 rpm in the large chainring. Ask your assistant to count pedal strokes for 15 seconds and multiply by 4—every minute. Ask your friend to record your heart rate every minute, and aim for an increase of 2–3 bpm during that period. Now, take it to the maximum. The test ends when you can't hold your cadence.

O'Reilly cites three training ranges: basic endurance (125 bpm to 80% of max), aerobic (80–90% of max), and anaerobic threshold, or AT (90% of max). Beginning in March, his plan calls for riders to train 10% in the anaerobic threshold range, 25–30% in the aerobic range, and 60–65% in the basic endurance range, a regimen that some people think easy but the coach says calls for discipline and concentration. He also uses a Polar Computer Interface that allows him to download workouts recorded by a number of commercial heart rate monitors to either an IBM compatible or an Apple computer. With this software you can graph a workout (time vs. heart rate), generate a bar graph in 10 bpm increments, and create tables of workout intensity over time. You can build a program around the results, starting with the maximum figure. More about the computer option later.

Whatever method you use to determine your MHR, remember that it's an important baseline used to determine your training parameters. So if you don't feel comfortable using any of these methods, get some help at your local health club.

Establishing ranges helps in a number of ways, whether you are an Olympian or a fitness cyclist. As you force yourself to stay in low gears during the early season, you'll also force yourself to stay in the basic endurance range, thus building a solid cardiovascular foundation and avoiding, if you wish, too many of what the enthusiasts call "junk miles." Please understand it is not a waste of time training below your target heart rate, except it won't build cardiovascular fitness, which is not necessarily bad. Sometimes you want to go out for an easy spin after a hard day.

Contrary to some notions about training, you don't burn more fat calories cycling below your target range. According to Dr. Steve Johnson, cycling for 1 hour at a heart rate of 120 bpm may burn 350 calories. Of these, about 175 may be fat calories. Conversely, if you pedal harder and get your heart rate to 160 bpm, you might burn 1,000 calories in an hour. At this intensity, only about one-fifth will be fat calories, but that still is 25 more (200) than the low-intensity ride. Dr. Johnson notes that when you ride below the target zone and burn a high percentage of fat calories, your body will replenish them first. To lose weight, it's best that you ride at the highest level you can comfortably sustain.

With the proper training, you can expect your AT level to rise during the season. Ned Overend, champion mountain biker, might have an AT level in the 150s in March but it can be in the 170s when he's peaking for a race. Likewise, your interval program should increase. For example, you might do five 3-minute intervals at 155 bpm in the spring and do the same set at 165 bpm in the summer after a training period. In effect, you've raised your AT and are getting better. On the other hand, if your AT goes down, you could be overtraining. Interval training is the secret to raising your AT. Longer intervals of 3–10 minutes are best for steady-rate riding while shorter training intervals of 30 seconds to 3 minutes best prepare you for riding that requires quick bursts of energy. But limit interval training to twice a week at the most. Too many cyclists still hold the notion that if it doesn't hurt, it's not really training. The fact is most beneficial results occur in a range where you are not hurting too much. And always remember that no coach talks about intervals and raising the AT without talking about rest. Skip Hamilton, who has coached Ned Overend and other champions, says there are two scenarios. "One is where you can't get your heart rate up. The other is when the workout level is so low and the perceived exertion is minimal, but your heart rate skyrockets. Either way, you're not in equilibrium. You need recovery."

You also need recovery if you wake up in the middle of the night with an accelerated heart rate, notice your home life is degenerating, feel you are heavy and ponderous on a bike, or find it difficult to recover from a hard ride.

Again, be your own coach. Read everything you can get your hands on, listen to the best advice you can find, but be your own coach. That will require you, above all, to listen to your body. If you're serious about cycling for health and fitness, you'll have to monitor the frequency, duration, and intensity of your riding. The first two are obvious; measuring intensity requires monitoring your heart rate either by counting your pulse or by using a heart rate monitor—and I recommend the latter, because it's much more precise. And as noted, you can get fancy and buy a multifunction heart rate monitor that will give you measurements you can download to your computer. Once you have an accurate measure of your target range, start to build a program within that range, taking into considering your cycling objective. If you plan to do long, steady mountain bike rides or century rides, then you can spend most of your time in the basic endurance and aerobic ranges; however, it's always useful to throw in some AT training because that is how you improve and, in turn, raise your AT level. Or if you're more comfortable with the target zones discussed in Chapter 5, that's fine. Use what works for you. The more you understand, monitor, and apply your heart rate, the better cyclist you'll be. In time you'll find a heart rate monitor just another piece of equipment you haul out before a ride. *Bicycling*'s editor Geoff Drake says, "I spend so much time wearing a heart rate monitor that sometimes I think I should have it surgically affixed." He's only half joking. Serious cyclists do have an attachment to this instrument because it's a sure-fire aid in becoming a better cyclist.

You will too.

See tables on pages 213, 215–216, 217, 219.

PEAKING

When I think of "peaks," I usually think of mountains, usually perfect in symmetry, a triangle with gently sloping sides. My first close-ups of a real mountain came when my ship would steam into Tokyo harbor and on a good day Mount Fuji, often with a snow cap, was in clear view. Then, Fuji was everywhere, from formal art to place mats, a symbol of pure and perfected nature that is so dear to the Japanese soul.

The image of the mountain resonates differently in different cultures but the meaning is similar. The mountain stands for challenge, achievement, something to be conquered. These days, however, "going to the mountaintop" has more to do with climbing than reflection, and climbers seem to bring more Coke cans than insights down from the summit.

An extended analogy pushed too far falls of its own weight, so I'll stop here. My point is that we should not think of our training as reaching the peak even though we might be climbing many mountains along the way. David Farmer, trainer to the mountain bike stars, including champions John Tomac and Juli Furtado, remarked in an interview, "What's most surprising is the ability to peak so frequently during one season. Somebody invented the myth that you can only peak so often. I don't know what sport that applies to, but it isn't mountain biking. Peaking situations can be spread out over an entire season. Juli proves that. For recreational riders, if you subject your body to fewer negatives—those things that push you beyond your limits, rather than holding you at them—you can perform more consistently."

Farmer emphasizes the importance of a heart rate monitor, even for a recreational athlete, and the need to establish season-long or year-round goals, whether to burn more fat, increase metabolic rate, or decrease fatigue. In Farmer's opinion, the "majority of sport riders have a pretty simple goal—to burn fat. And the body burns fat more efficiently at 65 to 75 percent of the maximum heart rate. But most mountain bikers, since the sport is so difficult, work at a higher intensity than they need to, at levels not conducive to burning fat."

In other words, if you cycle off-road 3–4 hours a week, you can get the most health benefits staying in the lower range. Hitting the hills hard every day, as many recreational riders do, will likely induce fatigue and burnout and put you in the anaerobic zone, which isn't the place to be to burn fat. You don't have to suffer the way the professional rider does. Having a training partner with shared goals will help you stay fresh and be able to respond to goals throughout the season.

Research is just beginning to catch up with mountain biking, a sport that requires so much focus and intensity it's easy for any rider to spend too much time in the anaerobic range. I'm referring to riding single tracks, not a Sunday in the park. On the other hand, road riding does give you time off—it's called freewheeling, and invites a different training regimen for the recreational rider. By midseason you'll likely be doing longer rides at faster speeds. First endurance, then speed, then endurance, then speed, and so on. Within the parameters of the advice already given, that might be enough for the fitness or fast recreational rider who is doing 150 miles a week and happy with it. No problem. But if you want to complete a century in five hours rather than six, do back-to-back centuries and participate in a club race, you can still put an edge on your fitness.

Here's some reassurance for the over-thirty crowd with a reasonable mileage base. Because, like most of us, you're probably pressed for time, Coach Walden recommends, "Go as hard as you can, as long as you can, and as often as you can. Within reason, it's hard to hurt mature riders. I call this 'pressure training.' I want you in the cooker. You only have so much time, so go right to your capacity. Deemphasize the technical training and just do it."

But for those who want to sharpen their skills, Walden has a few suggestions. Though he's a coach of road cyclists, the broad principles pertain to all cycling.

1. Most riders emphasize distance, then intensity. Try bringing up the intensity first. For example, if you want to ride 17 mph during a club event or century, train at 19 mph until you can't. When you're tired, don't slow down. Stop, rest, and get back to 19 mph. Intensity training will help you build endurance.
2. To build power for a set distance, such as a time trial, train at a higher speed than you can maintain. For example, if you want to do 20 miles in an hour, train at 23 mph and go as far as you can. Recover and rest until you can't do it any more. In time you'll be able to do the distance, in intervals, at a greater speed that you'd hoped to maintain.
3. To improve climbing, find two short, steep ascents with a valley in between, so you can work both sides of the street, as it were. On each hill mark a section of hundred yards. From a dead stop start climbing in an easy gear. When you reach the beginning of the hundred-yard mark, shift to a higher gear and accelerate. And when on top of that gear, shift to the next higher (smaller cog). Pedal easily to the top, descend, and start all over again on the other side.
4. To build speed, ride with a group and have designated riders lead out a sprint and the other riders must come around them. Do this drill into the wind. Or in a big gear.
5. The week before an event, cut down on endurance work and concentrate on speed. If Walden catches his riders forcing the pace two days before the event, he hits them with an old pump on the back of the head.
6. Walden defines cadence as revolutions per minute times pedal

pressure or "energy burn rate." Each of us has an ideal cadence, which is our most effective way of burning energy. The idea is to stay close to that cadence while handling the biggest gear possible.

For those truly interested in peak performance, take this test to discover your ideal cadence. You'll need a flat course, a cycle computer with speed and cadence functions, and a heart rate monitor. Needless to say, you should be in shape to do this.

1. Ride in about an 83-inch gear (52×17) at 22 mph. Note cadence and heart rate after it stabilizes. Recover.
2. Use the same course, distance, and speed but shift to the next highest gear (e.g. 52×16). Same procedure as in 1.
3. Repeat 2.
4. Repeat 3.

To check validity, reverse the order two days later. Do 2, and then 1. Two days later repeat at a slightly higher speed.

Analyze the number to find optimum cadence and gear at each speed. You'll find them by looking at the lowest heart rate at each of the speeds. For example, at 22 mph you might be more efficient at 85 rpm than at 90 rpm.

Walden doesn't suggest you do this for all your gears. He simply underscores the relationship between cadence and physiology and encourages us to use efficient gears that result in the lowest heart rate. There's no better way of becoming your own coach and trainer.

It's one thing to be watched by a coach, but entirely something else to watch yourself on videotape. And why not. The proliferation of video cameras makes self-coaching even more of a reality. In the old days, cyclists would pedal on stationary rollers in front of mirrors to examine and improve their cycling styles. Now we can watch ourselves on the road or trails in real time.

Ideal Cadence/Gear at 22 MPH

Gear (inches)	Speed (mph)	Cadence	Heart Rate (bpm)
Trial No. 1			
83	22	90	156–57
88	22	85	150–52
88	22	85	154–55
83	22	90	157–58
Trial No. 2			
88	22	85	152–53
83	22	90	158–60
83	22	90	159–61
88	22	90	154–55

Though we have looked at cycling from many angles, the angles are static. But bike size, fit, and use are dynamic and are best considered that way. To underscore the importance of this technique, every Olympic mountain and road bike prospect is videotaped, and the success of this technique has caused bike-riding camps and even clubs to use it as a training tool.

If you don't own a video camera, consider renting one. I recommend that cycling clubs rent a camera for a day and get maximum use from it. You'll learn more if the camera has a motorized lens and autofocus. A VCR with slow-motion and freeze-frame features is best. A tripod will help eliminate excessive motion. If you shoot from a car, someone else, of course, has to do the driving. Pick a road without traffic. A Sunday morning session has worked best for me.

Actually you might want to begin by having someone videotape you on an indoor trainer, so you can analyze bike fit and your basic riding position. Ideally, you'd be taped from the front, rear, and side as you pedal with hands on the drops at about 90 rpm. Bob Pritchard, who's company Somax does videotape motion analysis, has found a few obvious problems.

While filming from the rear, the most common problem was incorrect saddle height, usually too high, so the hips rock across the pedal stroke. Since most of us have one leg that's longer than the other, the videotape often picks up this discrepancy, showing the shorter leg dropping. In turn, the longer leg does more work. After the requisite analysis, the solution might be putting a shim of some kind under the heel of the shorter leg until it is even with the other. Runners frequently compensate for leg length discrepancy but cyclists, precisely because they can't see themselves in motion, rarely do.

From the front, watch the knees to determine whether one or both are moving sideways while pedaling, a common practice. If your knees fly outward, you might have to improve internal hip rotation by the "Z" stretch. Pritchard recommends that you "sit on the floor with one foot positioned on its side in front of your crotch and the other on its side behind you. Slowly bend forward and backward at the hips as far as possible."

On the other hand, to increase external rotation, "Lie on your back with the soles of your feet together and your knees as close to the floor as possible. Slide your feet away from your body, then pull them back in." Do this without raising your knees.

With a videotape of your side view, observe the maximum angle each knee opens to. Ideally, this should be 150 degrees. Stop the tape and measure. Also, look at the angle made by your elbow when on the drops. It should be 110 degrees.

At the Carpenter/Phinney Training Camp in Colorado, much of the riding is in the hills so the videotaping is done there. Connie Carpenter recommends filming in the hills because that's where the rider's habits tend to be exaggerated. Once the filming is done, the coaches look at the shoulders, arms, and hands to determine how relaxed the rider is. If you are not relaxed, your shoulder will likely be hunched, elbows locked, and grip tight. In Carpenter's words, "If you're not relaxed on the handlebar, you can't steer and can't react to a situation." That's why she and her husband, David, work so hard on relaxation because it makes riders more efficient, comfortable, and safe.

Now the coaches' focus shifts to climbing style. If I am rocking too much or pedaling frantically while climbing, I am probably in too low a gear. If I'm rocking from side to side, I'm likely pushing too big a gear. The same is probably true if I'm bobbing my head and using too much shoulder motion while climbing in the saddle.

The camera can tell me if I move heavily from being seated to the standing position, which will cause me to lose momentum. I should work on a smooth transition.

The video camera offers infinite possibilities, depending on your goals. If you want to hone your racing skills, you can be videotaped on- or off-road descending and taking corners. It's a tool that is bound to make you a more efficient rider and thereby improve your performance.

Ten years ago coaches held the secrets of your success. Now the keys are in your own hands. Heart rate monitors can tell the state of your fitness and from that number you can decide a training range. Cyclometers can measure mileage, cadence, elapsed time, elevation, and any combination of these. The video camera permits you to bring the ride home for analysis. Now computers allow you to store and analyze your training data. For example, Olympic cyclists at the Colorado Springs Training Center visit the exercise physiology lab after every ride and dump their training data into a computer. The computer, in turn, analyzes workouts, compares the day's session with a previous one, and charts future workouts.

The fast recreational or fitness rider might think computer training is overkill but that's not necessarily the case. For example, by charting a graph of your weekly mileage and average speed, you might be moved to new and higher goals. As noted earlier, you can analyze your heart rate at different cadences. Indeed, you can find the optimum cadence for all usable gears, something coaches of the past only dreamed about. Cycling software programs offer enormous potential, answering questions for which you could only guess the answer. For example, what might happen to my weekly average speed if I cut the time on my weekly 4-hour ride by 15 minutes? Given the results of my training rides, what is the best time I can hope for a century? And so on.

One of the most useful tools for the recreational cyclists is to buy a computer interface, mentioned earlier, that will allow you to record and then analyze your heart rate over time. The Vantage Performance Analysis is one on the market, but there will be many more before you read this. Since one of these units can cost $700, at this time it might be wiser for bike clubs to invest in the technology until the price comes down. (Consult *Bicycling* for the most up-to-date product reviews and information.)

Fortunately, there are many far less expensive products on the market. The BIKER software program for around $30 is adequate for recording mileage and time. But it can also display weekly to annual statistics and awards aerobic points depending on training. With the BIKER you can set mileage goals, and a bar graph will show how well you are progressing toward your goals.

This is just one example of the many commercial programs on the market that will help you become your own coach and truly contribute to peak performance. If you want complete nutritional information on all food, try Food Processor 11. You can plan a meal that best suits your physiological needs. If you want a weekly diet analysis, this program's for you.

If you'd rather not use our formula for determining gear inches, which really is a pain, consider GEARCART or GEAR CALCULATOR. Or if you'd rather do it yourself, consider using Lotus 1-2-3 for developing spread sheets to create a training log that includes weekly, monthly, and annual mileage totals. And so on.

Most of the commercial programs are available for IBM-compatible and Apple computers. Whatever you use, please give serious consideration to tracing your performance this way. Computers take the guesswork out of our training and force us to be mindful of the smallest detail.

Just when you think this book is becoming too technical, here is a reprieve. Computers can analyze your cycling but can't do the work for us. One area that has been given increased attention in all sports, including cycling, is "subliminal training," which, simply put, is the use of cues and hidden messages to change behavior. Gary Beale, Ph.D., who runs the Sierra Center for Peak Performance in Nevada, has brought subliminal training to cycling and creates personalized subliminal tapes containing positive statements about one's cycling process. He records the statements with music below the level of conscious hearing. The U.S. Cycling Federation has used the system successfully with junior riders. Though the jury is still out on this particular system, no athlete will deny the importance of relaxation, goal setting, and visualization.

And dreaming. Cheryl McLaughlin, Ph.D., contends that "champions excel because they think differently than other athletes," and she has translated this observation into a three-point plan to help all of us develop a winning mind-set. The first ingredient is having a dream, something that is exciting and fun to think about. Maybe you want to ride 20 miles in under an hour, do a century in under 6 hours, or finally clean every hill in that 10-mile stretch of single track.

When you have a dream, plan how you will make it come true. But don't be just a dreamer; give yourself long enough to execute it. Dr. McLaughlin encourages realism, adding that most athletes expect too much too soon. Then, list all the steps needed to make it happen. If you dream about climbing better, you might have to lose ten pounds, which means you might have to eat less pizza and drink less beer. Whatever the steps, put them on paper or in your computer.

Finally, devise the daily workout schedule that will make your dream come true. To do an across-the-Rockies mountain bike ride two years from now, you might want to substantially increase your upper body strength, which will probably call for a weight program. And above all, be an optimist. Most champions are. They believe in themselves.

There is an inner game of cycling, though not fully documented. Cyclists talk about being one with the bike or sensing that the bike disappears beneath them. The inner game might be marked by a feeling of lightness on the pedals, a kind of exuberance when hill climbing, an invincibility. The game might mean doing endless, playful rounds of speed work and not being fatigued or the sometimes dangerous dream states that cross-country racers experience. The game, if projected against a screen, would be three-dimensional: you, the bike, and the space you glide through all acting with and on each other, sometimes in indescribable ways. Cyclists report feeling this as they glide through nature, taking part of it along as memory and goal. I'm not sure how this works but I can remember seeing a large fox in the Scottish Highlands who ran parallel to my bike route for a mile. Strange as it might seem, I was a fitter, better, more technically astute cyclist for that distance. At least I felt that way. I'm sure a videotape would have shown me tooling along, weary on the ninth day of a 10-day trip. I recall on the same trip cycling the tight lanes of Cornwall with a friend and smelling smells I had not sensed since I was a child growing up in England. And what was that earthy, swampy, moss smell about shoulder high that greeted us of a morning? Perhaps because cyclists move through space and over varied terrains the universe works on us in strange ways. I'm not just talking about speed. Most sports have that. I'm talking about being inside cycling and at the same time being inside the space and the moments one cycles through. I don't mean spaced out; I mean spaced "in"—having a consciousness of what one passes through.

For me, the inner game of cycling comes when all other games are over. The bike fits, is light, and in proper pitch. I am riding smart on a good day alone or with friends. Perhaps I have made love in the morning. Now all the how-to information I have worn like an anchor drops from me like sweat but comes back subtly to police my movements. This game, I'm convinced, is at the other side of coaching when not only is your body willing, but the mind is willing too, accepting all the good advice then cycling through it to find the ecstasy beyond. Surely at the center of this inner game is play, a touch of abandon, a hint of the child.

So, in that spirit, let me offer a coda to this chapter. I've been listening to expert advice for more than a decade and am getting a little tired of it. You know, one Olympic coach after the other telling us to do this and that. I mean, cycling is supposed to be fun, remember? All right, while I'm not going to suggest you ditch the training program, I will suggest you ease your grip on the handlebars just a little.

For me, cycling is most rewarding when I make it a significant part of my life, such as in commuting, when I become free of my car. I know I'm supposed to ride with others but I have so much fun riding by myself, chasing my shadow. As I cruise along the country roads of Pennsylvania, I like to do speed work or fartlek, as the experts call it, to break the lull. I might sprint to a farmhouse, past a reliably angry dog, or in concert with the rare Burma-Shave signs. I don't know that I'm working, let alone getting my heart rate up, but the monitor says otherwise. I keep speed work on the edge of play and can end the game anytime I want.

For no particular reason, all this reminds me of professional coach Mike Neel, who grew up training horses and has a decidedly visceral approach to training cyclists, depending more on his feel for the riders than strictly on scientific measurement. Some coaches speak of peaking, as if you are the shape coming from the putty. Neel might say, "You need to let your form come. Tease it. All of a sudden you'll be riding, doing the same thing you've done for days and you think: 'I'm going to go hard today.' You put it in the big ring and go, and you sustain it. Then you say, 'My God, I guess I'm getting fitter.' That's the way it should be. From then on, you do it every time because you've been patient."

Neel's a minimalist, rejecting odometers and aerobars, which he calls "jungle-gym bars." He likes the "pure, simplistic, beautiful bike." And now that we have loaded ourselves up with all the right stuff, Neel's words serve as a fitting reminder that it's the bike we sit on. No need to become a Christmas tree.

I get lost often but probably not often enough. Fast recreational rides or races are usually just that, stiff rides from point-to-point, nose on the stem, hands on the drops. So much is missed that way. To put more fun in the sport, get lost on purpose or throw away the map once in a while. This is usually easier to do off-road but important for any rider.

Be careful with this one but don't be afraid to play the fool. Test your skills. Ride without hands, telling yourself you're checking the frame alignment. Dodge spots on the road or trail, play tag with a companion, or practice your track stands. I do this at stoplights but try to make sure there is a pole handy just in case my skill deceives me. If you're on the road, by all means watch for traffic.

133

Conduct business on your bike. Golfers do it, so why not cyclists? My supervisor and I try to conduct most of our business during a bike ride (or a run). I won't hazard a guess at the psychological ramifications, but I think meetings conducted this way are open and honest. One is able to "cut to the chase" more quickly. And unlike with golf, it's all right to get to the top of the hill before your boss.

Instead of a heart rate monitor or a cyclometer being a slave, make it an instrument of play. Within reason, bounce back and forth between two numbers (heart rate or mph) and watch the complexion of the ride change.

If you are primarily a road rider, get on a mountain bike, even if you have to borrow one. The mountain bike invites play, bunny hopping, bouncing around, jumping curbs and logs, and falling down. Conversely, if you are primarily a mountain biker, ride a road bike to appreciate its simplicity, geometry, and speed. Mix up your miles.

Get a tandem and take your spouse, friend, lover, or child along for a ride.

Though I've previously emphasized planning before a ride, discard that advice and decide to ride on the spur of the moment. Call a friend and have him or her decide the destination. Sometimes I hook up with a solitary rider and ask the cyclist if he or she wants company. Careful with this tactic. You could finish a long way from home.

To break your training regimen, consider riding at night, which is perfectly acceptable if you have a light and wear reflective clothing.

Conventional wisdom calls you to push yourself. Try to peak, taper, and peak again. Pick rides in May, July, and September, and try to peak for those instead of looking for that one season high.

Stop and stop again. I won't repeat the "smelling the roses" slogan but will say that some of my most memorable moments on long tours were when I stopped. Even on short rides with friends. I'm surprised at how open men are to talking to other men, in particular, during a lull in the ride. Defenses are down and the heart speaks.

Candace Burnswick of Oakdale, New York, has a very simple mantra: "Many miles, equals many smiles, equals peace." And she got there the hard way as she started riding to kick a substance abuse habit. Cycling on- and off-road helps her remember why it's so good to be alive and makes her feel like a kid again. For her, the "sweet spot" is "smelling the first bloom of spring, the quietness of riding through the snow, the sounds of the birds. Cycling is the best natural high."

When you are in the groove, cycling is more than keeping the heart rate in the right zone or recovering in record time. Peak performance is, indeed, climbing to the mountaintop and bringing home just a little soul.

CROSS-TRAINING

Few cyclists don't cross-train. Even the ones who ride every day usually lift weights, jump rope, or do t'ai chi. In truth, the term "cross-training" is a misnomer, suggesting one has to reach for it, cross over, and taste a sport that's a distance from the core activity. Cross-training is really enlightened training in the best sense of the word because the practice will help train, condition, and teach the entire body. And not insignificantly, cross-training will probably keep you injury-free.

Without redlining the fact, we have been talking about cross-training throughout this book. In effect, when I suggest riding a road bike to develop cadence and spin and the mountain bike to develop upper body strength and hand-eye coordination, I'm really talking about cross-training. Having both bikes in your arsenal will ensure that you enjoy a full season of cycling and in the process develop a variety of on-bike skills.

STRENGTH TRAINING

As I write this chapter, I'm flipping through 300 questionnaires from recreational cyclists who have outlined their training in some detail. Of the 300, only about 10 said they rode their bikes all year and didn't do any other exercise. Of these, most live in Florida and California. No surprise here. I personally know no serious cyclist who does not engage in some kind of serious cross-training—and I don't mean just in the so-called off-season. All the editors at *Bicycling* practice some kind of cross-training, be it running, Rollerblading, cross-country skiing, and the like. Few road and mountain bike racers don't swap bikes sometime during the year. Though cycling is my primary fitness activity, I practice cross-training year-round, adding running and free weights to my schedule. I'm particularly enamored of the stair climber, which has made me stronger in the hills on my bike and a fairly good runner with relatively few miles a week. Knock on wood, I've never had a serious overuse injury during my ten years of cross-training. The preponderance of cyclists I interviewed for this book usually migrate to other exercises in the late fall and winter but all ride either a stationary bike or some kind of a mountain bike. Most, even in the warmer climates, follow the swing of the seasons, suggesting, among other things, that there is a psychological benefit to backing off from a primary sport and getting recharged by practicing a complementary activity. By February, most cyclists are restless to get on the road, exactly how I feel as I write these words looking out at the twenty inches of snow covering my farm.

In reviewing the questionnaires from recreational cyclists, what surprised me was not that almost 100 percent of the respondents practiced cross-training, but that they did it in such a willy-nilly way. No criticism intended; I know willy-nilly. Perhaps this is due to the focus and organization the cycling season requires. In the off-season why not just get the heart rate up, burn some calories, and have a good time because come spring you'll be outside where the real work begins. That's a fair and sensible proposition, one that I can readily embrace. However, few recreational cyclists interviewed seem to feel that the nonbike training contributed much to their fitness, and many reluctantly accepted that they would be overweight by spring by an average of ten pounds.

Given the demands of life, you might be completely happy with doing a little of this and a little of that, just to keep the blood circulating. But if you want to improve your cycling, perhaps a more structured program is in order. My comments notwithstanding, I was particularly struck by the remarks of Fredric Richter of Annville,

Pennsylvania, who rides his windtrainer while watching boxing on television, adding that the three minutes of intense activity followed by a minute of rest suits him just fine. (Actually, I've followed a similar regimen except I hit the heavy bag during the bout. I can hardly raise my hands by the tenth round.)

In addition to providing a needed respite from a demanding sport, cross-training can actually help isolate cycling-specific muscles and work them harder with less effort. And as a further benefit, cross-training can help reduce overuse injuries which, though not the bane of cyclists, can still be a problem. And as every athlete knows, you do get stale exercising in the same mode so variety definitely has a positive psychological effect.

Steve Johnson, Ph.D., suggests that this regimen can "improve performance by conditioning muscles not normally involved in your sport. This is especially true for aerobic sports in which inactive skeletal muscles may contribute to performance by helping remove the lactic acid produced by their active counterparts. A recent study demonstrated that upper body aerobic training can enhance the aerobic performance of the lower body by reducing the accumulation of lactic acid during lower body exercise. So maybe swimming can help your cycling."

An example closer to home, as Dr. Johnson acknowledges, is weight training whether through circuit training or with free weights. Few serious recreational cyclists don't lift weights, especially in the off-season. Richard Lamphier of Elk Rapids, Michigan, rides about 25,000 miles a year and uses a "torture chamber" at home and his local Y for leg presses, leg extensions, and leg curls. Tony Mourkas of Hampden, Maine, does circuit training at least three times a week out of season and shares this regimen with tens of thousands of cyclists who have made high-repetition circuit training a mainstay of their fitness program. In fact, the medical literature is rich with data that suggests strength training is important for cyclists. Many coaches and physiologists now believe that weight training is absolutely essential if cyclists are to reach their potential. Harvey Newton, an instructor at the University of Colorado, noted that rarely "do cyclists possess levels of strength and power equal to their skill." His research has shown that "there are numerous benefits to a progressive resistance training program including: gains in strength, development of power, increases in muscular endurance and prevention and rehabilitation of injuries."

Newton differentiates between cardiovascular (endurance) and strength circuits, recommending the former be used during the first 2–4 weeks of off-season training, serving as a kind of bridge. The cardiovascular circuit offers little rest between stations, high repetitions, lower weights, and five to ten times through the circuit. A good rule of thumb is to allow 20–40 seconds for each exercise with a short recovery time in between. Conversely, a strength circuit training regimen would offer more rest between stations, fewer repetitions, higher weights, and three to five times through the circuit.

My company, Rodale Press, Inc., offers the cardiovascular circuit every morning at 7 A.M., and it's clear to me that I get a better workout under supervised conditions. Sometimes I do a modified circuit training at home, skipping rope between high-repetition sets with free weights, but it's not the same, primarily because I don't have the stations, especially for leg work—and that is what should be emphasized in the off-season. A variety of multipurpose home gyms are available which offer a more than adequate training. The objective of circuit training is to work different parts of the body. For example, my program after warm-up starts by exercising the arms and shoulders, then the abdomen, legs, and trunk, usually with high repetitions (10–15). If I'm doing progressive sets, I'll increase the weight slightly on the second set, doing fewer repetitions. Most programs call for at least two circuits of 10–12 exercises, which should take about 40 minutes. Some cyclists prefer doing basic circuit training Monday and Friday and a progressive circuit on Wednesday.

Circuit training will increase your strength, help maintain your cardiovascular conditioning, and work areas of the body not normally touched while cycling. Coaches often recommend for racers a 4-week period of circuit and cross-training activities as a bridge from a strenuous cycling season to a strength-training phase, thus reducing the chance of injuries.

While circuit training will certainly do no harm and will contribute to your overall fitness, some coaches and trainers at the Olympic Training Center in Colorado Springs no longer recommend that racers engage in circuit training during the off-season. Though long a staple of the United States Cycling Federation's training program, of late circuit training has been shown to have fewer cardiovascular benefits than were once thought. The sentiment these days at the training facility is to eschew circuit training and, after the bridge period, get into strength training. I won't argue with established, reliable research. However, I've personally known hundreds and communicated with thousands of recreational cyclists who have used circuit training primarily as an off-season activity with good results. While circuit training, per se, doesn't have much of a carryover effect to your cycling, it will likely make the upper body stronger. However, it can serve as a transitional activity as you move from bike riding to a full-fledged weight program. Then if you want a weight-training regimen that specifically impacts your cycling, a more traditional program is in order.

To summarize, you might begin a transitional weight-training program in October for 4 weeks using light weights and high repetitions 2–3 times a week. Circuit training, as described, would serve this purpose. It's important that the muscles get used to lifting.

The next phase is a preliminary 4–6-week period involving 3 weekly workouts. Customarily you'd do 8–12 repetitions of each exercise and 4 sets.

Exercises that are particularly useful for cyclists include the step-up. You step up on a bench with a barbell on your back, safely working the quadriceps. The traditional bench press is a great way to strengthen the cyclist's typically weak upper body. Sit-ups or, better still, crunchers will help alleviate back problems. Leg presses will increase quad strength. And the barbell row will improve arm and shoulder strength.

With this base you are ready for 4–6 weeks of strength training using 4 or more sets of each exercise with no more than 8 repetitions. During the last month of this period, you concentrate on a cycling-specific weight program, particularly leg presses, step-ups, and lunges.

CLIMBING

The old division between aerobic and strength athletes has finally crumbled. Research has shown that increased leg strength will increase your VO_2 max, your body's oxygen-carrying capacity. Moreover, weight training will help even out the customary differences in strength between the right and left legs and balance the strength of the opposing quadriceps and hamstrings.

By the way, don't put away your heart monitor when you are doing your strength training, which is best done in the 160–180 bpm range, depending on your age. Allow your heart rate to drop to 102 bpm between sets.

Though strength training is an essential part of my off-season regimen, it's not my favorite. That title belongs to the stair climber, available in almost all gyms and health clubs, which is becoming very popular with cyclists because it so closely approximates the cycling motion. When cycling you move around on the bike. Climbing a hill you might be out of the saddle pushing off on the balls of the feet. For power you're sitting back in the saddle working the backs of the legs and the gluteus maximus. You can approximate the same cycling positions on a stair climber and at the same time vary the pedal height and the number of strokes per minute. For example, you can replicate a 90-rpm cycling cadence and run your heart rate into the target zone as if you were on a bike.

Hank Lang, a colleague and Vermont coach, is one of the nation's foremost authorities on cross-training, advising many triathletes and world and Olympic champions in many sports. He is enthusiastic about the stair climber and offers a specific program for the cyclist in training and the recreational rider. See the accompanying table.

	Cyclist in Training	Recreational Rider
Monday	Off	Off
Tuesday	Steps: 45+ min.; WI = 5 × 3 min., Level 4; RI = 2–3 min., Level 1	Steps: 45+ min.; pyramid intervals; WI = 1-2-3-4-3-2-1, Level 3; RI = 2 min., Level 2
Wednesday	Bike: 1 hr.; Levels 1–2	Bike: 45+ min., Levels 1–2; Pickups = 30 sec.; RI = 3 min.
Thursday	Steps: 30 min., Level 2; Pickups = 1 min.; Level 3; RI = 4–5 min.	Steps: 30 min., Level 2; Small steps, vary body position

Much as I like stair climbers and use them religiously, not everyone has access to these machines or chooses to use them. One of the most popular forms of cross-training for cyclists is still running, which for most means a workout three times a week for a distance of 3–5 miles. Frank Shorters reminds us that if you use running as part of an off-season regimen, think about it aerobically. That is, you are running not to break records or prepare for a marathon, but to maintain a basic level of fitness without putting yourself at orthopedic stress, something cyclists are not used to. Only if you want to punish yourself, consider this workout recommended by some cycling coaches: Run uphill on a hiking trail for 30–50 minutes twice a week. When you feel you've mastered the terrain, add a weight belt or a backpack filled with rocks. Of course, you won't be able to do much running but you'll get a tremendous workout. Unless you're masochistic, I'd

---

Key

A cyclist in training is someone who rides 5–6 days per week in season, averaging 100–150 miles per week.

A recreational rider is a more casual cyclist who rides 3–4 times per week in season, averaging 40–100 miles, in addition to participating in other sports.

WI = work interval; RI = rest interval

For instance, "WI = 5 × 3 min., Level 4; RI = 2–3 min., Level 1," means you should do five 3-minute work intervals at Level 4 intensity interspersed with 2–3-minute rest intervals at Level 1 intensity.

Pickups are short, high-rpm cycling intervals designed to develop leg speed. These lack the formality of structured work and rest intervals. Instead, do them spontaneously when you feel rested and ready.

Intensity Levels

This intensity scale details how hard you should exercise throughout the program. It's based on four factors: type of work, percentage of maximum heart rate, a subjective rating of effort on a 10-point scale (perceived exertion or PE), and an approximation of how long you could sustain each intensity. For instance, if the schedule calls for a Level 3 workout, simply refer to the four factors to determine the intensity. This scale is appropriate for endurance training only.

---

pass on the rocks. I'd recommend you run for the aerobic value and don't try to make a simple workout complex. On the other hand, I run all year, more in the winter, and have never found running to hurt my cycling. Though I do my share of running intervals and fartlek, what I consider essential to my cycling is running the hills, which strengthens my quadriceps and seems to carry over directly to my cycling. And I cycle with a lot of runners, and though they tend to grind big gears, they are usually very powerful. So used as an adjunct to cycling, running is a great off-season choice.

Everyone has a favorite off-season activity. Coach Mike Walden is no exception. He is not an advocate of weight training or of running, which he thinks causes too many injuries. His advice: Don't do anything with your legs that doesn't mimic the motion of riding a bike. He is a fan of mountain biking, cross-country skiing, and speed skating, a sport with a long history of developing athletes who excelled in cycling—Sheila Young-Ochowicz in particular. The reason for the high crossover is that speed skaters use the same muscles as cyclists.

Walden divides the off-season into capillary and muscle development periods. The first refers to a low-intensity period, usually about a month, during which you would ride a fixed gear bike at a heart rate of less than 135 bpm or about two-thirds of your maximum, with allowances given for age. (Many cyclists convert an old beater bike to a fixed gear by combining a chainring of 42 with a cog that has 13, 14, 15, or 16 teeth, which gives a gear inch range of 70–90 inches, which will allow you to ride at 80–90 rpm.) This might seem like old school to you, and it is, but many cyclists swear by fixed-gear riding, claiming that it improves their cadence and other skills while gently building base mileage. Walden likes his road cyclists to ride at least 1,000 miles in a fixed gear before spring training.

In truth, this "capillary" period during which the body does low-intensity activities is recommended by many coaches and trainers I know. It gives the body the opportunity to rest and recover before the muscle development stage begins. Instead of weight training, Walden (and others) recommends cross-country skiing, skating, or hill walking, a curious though effective exercise in which one climbs, and descends, and traverses a hill, ideally one that is soft underfoot and shaped like a bowl. This is done as hard and fast as possible for an hour, three times a week. Add hand weights later on.

In the off-season most cyclists change the duration, frequency, and

145

intensity of their exercise, sometimes drastically. For example, I will cut back on all three elements, especially intensity. I simply don't want to train as hard, for both physiological and psychological reasons. Others replicate the same intensity in compatible exercises such as cross-country skiing. Longtime professional racers Greg LeMond and Andy Hamsten for years used cross-country skiing to balance an extremely demanding race schedule, without losing any aerobic advantage. LeMond acknowledges that "Even when your technique is not that good, you can still get a good workout. Your heart rate is always at 160 to 170 beats per minute." Skating is all the more attractive to cyclists since the "skating" technique was introduced a few years ago to top American amateur and professional cyclists.

No chapter on cross-training or off-season fitness is complete without some mention of the indoor resistance trainer, perhaps the most maligned piece of exercise equipment ever to grace a basement or bedroom. I didn't have to conduct extensive research to know that most people consider this form of cycling boring, equating it with watching paint dry. Whatever kind of resistance trainer you own—and there's a ton on the market, including the ones you can hook up your road bike to—don't sell short this training device, which is useful when it rains or snows, or when your schedule is tight. Just don't ask too much of it.

Cycling at a 20-mph pace for an hour at a high resistance setting will burn 1,133 calories, which is nothing to sneeze at. But most people aren't able to stay on their bikes that long. I know a friend who sits in front of the television on his trainer for a football game, approximately three hours. At the rate he pedals, he is cycling well below his target zone and not doing much good at all. He is better off working harder for shorter periods. As on the bike, you should plan specific workouts for your indoor trainer. By now you know the drill: Wear your heart monitor, which will make indoor time quality time. Mix up your program as you would outdoors. One day do a 50-minute workout at 75 percent of your maximum heart rate. Another day do intervals. Cycle for 60 seconds at about 90 percent of maximum, recover to 70 percent, and repeat. Do 2–3 sets of 3–5 intervals with recovery in between. You can vary your interval program to meet your training needs. Another day you might want to do short-duration intervals at maximum resistance for 15 seconds and recover to 65 percent. Do this for 20–25 minutes with a 10-minute warm-up and cooldown. Other days should be for rest or aerobic activities such as skiing or mountain biking.

The challenge for most indoor cyclists is not reaching 90 percent of maximum heart rate but just staying on the damn machines. To help allay boredom, have a plan or program each time you sit in the indoor saddle. Most people enjoy listening to loud music. Use a fan to help control your body temperature and this, in turn, will make your cycling more efficient. Or if you want to invest in one of those expensive stationary trainers with computers, you can race indoors against the best cyclists in the world, though you might not want to.

Let me close this chapter with some examples from the real world. These people work, have children, go to school, and try to keep fit in the process.

1. John G. Seiler of St. Cloud, Minnesota, reports that 3–4 days a week he spends 20 minutes on upper-body weight lifting and 10 minutes on a stair climber. One day a week he spends 25 minutes on a treadmill. He sneaks out on his mountain bike during those sunny January and February days.

2. Linda Herrick of Binghamton, New York, rides the wind-trainer and devours great books. If the book is really great, she'll ride longer. She does this every day except when she practices t'ai chi.

3. Merle Glines of Paris, Maine, rides the Schwinn Air Dyne daily for 30 minutes, cross-country skis, and backpacks. However he trains, he feels great in the spring. By late June he feels even better and by late August feels like racing anyone within 20–25 years of his age group.

4. John DeFayette of Schuyler Falls, New York, skis, snowshoes, and works out 3 times a week on Lifecycle, Concept II rower, Stair Stepper, Downhill Ski Machine, and weights. He gets out on his mountain bike on occasion.

5. Chris Etue, of Saint Marys, Ontario, runs 2–3 times a week,

cross-country skis daily, and uses a windtrainer 2–3 times a week with intervals. She uses a heart rate monitor to raise her anaerobic threshold and decrease her recovery time. She also plays ice hockey.

6. William Melton of Rockville, Maryland, admits to no off-season. He rides year-round if the ground is not icy or snow-covered. If the weather is bad for 3–4 consecutive days, he gets on his stationary bike.

7. John Bates of Saint Louis, Missouri, uses the Cyclosimulator by Cateye and cycles every other day about 350 miles a month. His program:

5 miles at 0% incline in 52×14 or 13 gear in about 12 minutes (warm-up)

5 miles at 1% incline in 52×14 or 13 gear in about 12.5 minutes

5 miles at 1% incline in 52×13 gear in about 13 minutes

5 miles at 2/1% incline in 52×41/13 in about 14 minutes

5 miles cooldown

8. K. C. Bailey of Mount Morris, New York, weight-trains 3 days a week from November through February: bench press, curls, leg lifts, hamstring lifts, and 100 sit-ups on the incline bench. He does 6 sets, 15 repetitions. He also uses the NordicTrack 3 days per week for 30–45 minutes, does easy cycling 1–3 days a week, Rollerblades 1–3 days a week if roads are clear, and does 500 crunches per day year-round. Since using the NordicTrack, he hasn't put on weight during the winter.

9. Marjorie Henderson of Huberdeau, Quebec, bought a windtrainer and keeps it in the kitchen, which is a good reminder. She uses it almost every day. It made a huge difference when she did her first road ride in the spring.

10. David Donly of Battle Creek, Michigan, cites work as his program. He lifts hundred-pound bags all day, sometimes more than 4,000 bags in a day. He walks his dog and cleans house. He cycles to work, though the deep snow is a challenge. He admits the snow and ice help with handling skills.

148

He doesn't own a car and enjoys equally his friends' praise and admonition.

Cross-training crosses geography and psychology. At the end of the season, the music changes and we dance to a less hectic beat. No cyclist I've interviewed does nothing during this period. Most mix and match exercises that suit their fashion. Neither rain, nor snow, nor dark of night can stop some cyclists; they ride year-round, often with a virtuousness that is unmistakable. Most people seem to have a go at the target zone and come March are none the worse for it. Some of us revel in fantasy. Tim Driscoll of Grand Forks, North Dakota, imagines that he rides his windtrainer while he counts the days until spring arrives. I am more enamored of this story than the one about the cyclist who locked himself in a dark closet and rode his stationary bike for 3-hour clips. Cycling should contribute to mental health, not detract from it. Give me North Dakota anytime. The cyclist who has a sense of humor during a weather- or psychology-inspired off-season will survive to ride another day. By all means, if you can stand a structured program as outlined here, do it and celebrate in the spring. If for you this time is play, stretch your legs to the music and move in whatever circles you circumscribe.

Level	Type of Work	% Max HR	PE	Hold For
1	Warm-up, recovery, easy distance	<70	1–3	2+ hrs.
2	Endurance, distance	70–80	3–7	1+ hrs.
3	Threshold, pace, easy intervals	80–90	6–8	1/2–1 hr.
4	Max VO$_2$, hard intervals, hill reps	85–95	8–9	5–20 min.
5	Anaerobic power, sprints	90–100	9–10	<3 min.

WEIGHT LOSS

I have a cyclist friend who is rotund, tubular, plump, and round. The Lycra jersey doesn't fit him so his gut is exposed every time he raises his arms above the shoulders. What he does to a pair of Lycra shorts is nobody's business. Yet he's a strong cyclist, able to put together back-to-back centuries. Sitting in behind him on the flat is like occupying a seat behind the lead engine on a fast train, so powerful is his pull. Though he considers hills anathema and will significantly increase his mileage to avoid elevation, he's a reasonably fit, healthy cyclist.

Go to any century ride, MS event, or organized tour, and you'll see more body types than listed in a physiology book. Like me, you might wonder how a certain bulbous individual can possibly ride a hundred miles but ride it he does. Now go to the start of a 10K run or marathon and witness the lean, Lycra-clad runners who look emaciated. Is there something about cycling that attracts heavy people? Well, yes and no.

One leitmotiv for this book is that cycling meets us at our level of need—and sometimes that need is very great. You have seen examples of people who can't walk or run but can pedal a bike. Or individuals who have the use of one leg and somehow manage to keep the cranks turning, suggesting that desire is a powerful muscle. We all know people who can't run because of knee, foot, or weight problems but readily take to the bike. Yes, cycling does embrace all those yearning to be fit. This democratic pull is yet another reason for its popularity.

151

ARCHETYPAL STORIES

Dorothy Tobe of Denver, Colorado, gained 10 pounds a year over a five-year period and had visions of herself as a "176-pound, middle-aged woman with varicose veins and diabetes, which runs in the family." So she cut out alcohol and junk food and got back on her Huffy bicycle, purchased at a K mart when she lived in rural Ohio. Soon she graduated to a Trek road bike she named Vishnu, the preserver god in Hindu mythology.

Through cycling and good nutrition, she lost more than 50 pounds in 6 months and decided to test her fitness by participating in an MS 150 (miles), which she completed successfully. Dorothy notes that she "had MS Tour teammates who used the tour to meet their own physical challenges whether it was part of their weight-loss program or simply an event to train for in their fitness regimen.

"In looking back to my obese days, the person I was then would never have imagined herself where she is today. I can attest to the advantages of being physically fit, whether it be the joy of eating or the joy of sex. Even my tired, painful legs disappeared, and I'd thought I was doomed to wear support hose for the rest of my life. The new awareness of my body has promoted awareness in mind, heart, and soul. Because of bicycling, I am more alert and happier (when I'm stressed or mad, I find some hills to attack). The confidence I gained in riding a bike, especially after surviving some frightening mountain bike downhills, has transferred to areas of life where I now will try new activities or ideas. Every time someone describes me as slender, I have bicycling to thank for saving me from the fetters of obesity."

This story, in addition to being a poignant reminder of the value of cycling for weight loss, is also a striking example of what I like to call the psychology of weight loss through cycling. The epiphany is usually a looking in the mirror or a realization of what the future might hold. Then a memory of youth when the bicycle was prominent in the imagination. Then the trip to the garage or basement to find a K mart special that doesn't resonate with "health", so one upgrades to a Trek, which in this instance is the Hindu god Vishnu, the Preserver of Life, so christened by the cyclist Tobe.

But as mortal men and women, we need goals, and the MS 150 has served as a stimulus for hundreds of thousands of health-conscious cyclists who wanted to contribute to a good cause while doing themselves a favor. That has proved a powerful combination. Fortunately the ride never ends with the completion of a trip, for the bike does more than shed weight; it allows us to develop a perspective—often a soulful perspective—on life. We see things more clearly and experience them more deeply. We are engaged. Sex, food, and relations become more precious. Our hunger and thirst for all things is heightened.

I am describing an archetypal story that I have witnessed or heard about a thousand times. Does this make cycling better than other sports? No, of course not; just different. It's different because it has a social dimension, takes us through space and time, and lets us explore environments in the process. The vast mobility cycling offers heightens the experience and transforms the participant. And if this is pop psychology, it comes from the heart and is born of deep experience and wonder about this sport.

Those of us who are blessed with the ability to move fast can't always appreciate the angst of a person who celebrates his or her life in slow time. Take Greg Wilson of Virginia, who was 200 pounds when he graduated from high school about ten years ago. On a frame of 5' 8", he felt the weight too much and could see himself leveling off at 250 pounds. The angel who appeared was in the guise of a cycling friend who encouraged Greg to ride but always left him in the dust. Still, no matter how much the angel laughed or how high the hills were, Wilson persevered. He bought a new bike, helmet, gloves, and speedometer, completing some stiff 70-mile hilly rides on the Blue Ridge Parkway. Through cycling and weight training, he dropped to 150 pounds. Since that time he has become something of a mountain man, completing the Assault on Mount Mitchell and climbing the steep Grandfather Mountain in Virginia. As you read this, he should be cycling the actual Tour de France race route. Not bad for a fat kid.

Greg Wilson's story is remarkable but not exceptional. I take nothing away from his marvelous feats to say that his accomplishments are within the grasp of everyone. Cycling accepts us in all our weighty splendor. The gearing comforts you on those long, arduous hills that embarrass one's fitness. The bike is your metaphor, always a little out front, going faster than you think you can or should. You wonder: How does this 25-pound frame support me so wistfully? With every turn of the pedals, the bicycle becomes closer to you; the ownership is more personal. The right bike is smooth, light, and fast and you want to become that. The law of mechanics says you will go faster at less weight but that is only half of it. Most of us are not magicians and must improve by painful increments. Cycling is incremental, allowing you to pile modest success upon success where in other sports you might be discouraged or even disenfranchised owing to injury or lack of progress. Weight loss through cycling is not just a transfer of energy from food, to you, to the drive train and to the pedals. To lose weight, you must enjoy the activity enough that you can stay on the bike long enough in the appropriate heart rate zone to ensure calorie consumption and weight loss. You must find pleasures and objectives that soon supersede the original goal of weight loss, as important as that might be. Cycling must enter your psychology on a cellular level so you can embrace the activity as a lifesport and not just a mechanical means of weight reduction. No one has fully explained or described what it means to "be in the groove" while cycling. To be sure it does mean that the bike fits perfectly and the ride has a quality of perfection. Moreover, when you are in the groove, you will feel a kind of transcendence, not in the religious sense, but in the sense that the body hovers above the bike as it sings along at speed. During this kind of ride you are "in" and "out" of nature constantly. I recall on some particularly exhilarating stretches in the Scottish Highlands a very distinct, unique heather plant, a certain sheep that stood out, the cut of a hillside all the while flying through countryside rich, green, and generic. Cycling invites good peripheral vision and the exactness of the camera lens. It is a way of seeing the world in slow time even though you might be dropping through a mountain pass at 40 mph. The culture of cycling is not so much marked by the beautiful patches people wear at cycling conventions, commemorating their other adventures, but by the private and public visions and reveries that invade our consciousness as we ride. Many people have told me about cycling giving them a different perspective on life. I don't just mean that cycling relaxed them so they could think more evenly about life. What I believe these cyclists meant was that cycling helped them deal with life more concretely, more specifically, perhaps even more metaphorically. I'll stop short of making poets out of bike riders, yet something happens on the road. I ride with friends who spend all week worshipping or chasing the numbers but come Sunday morning deep into a ride the language changes and they talk of dreams, seek out blooming dogwood trees, and wonder about death. Men who don't touch their fathers in conversation during the week have done so in my company under the influence of this soft, rhythmic, beguiling sport called cycling.

I am talking to you about weight loss within a compelling context because that is how cyclists have talked to me. Weight loss is often the banner that begins the ride but quality of life is often writ larger at the end. Take Gary Madine of Allentown, Pennsylvania, who three years ago weighed 208 pounds on a 5' 9" frame, couldn't button his pants; had slightly high cholesterol, borderline high blood pressure, and an unusually high resting pulse; and suffered from extreme stress and other ailments. All in all, very much like the archetypal twentieth-century man. Once a cyclist of sorts, he found marriage, home ownership, fatherhood, a stressful job, and childcare worries seemed to take the activity out of his reach. He was down to cycling eighteen miles a year. Gary had to hold his breath while tying his shoes because his stomach was so large. He concluded his condition ridiculous and decided to do something about it: commute to work on his bike. On his first commute, he says, "My heart felt as if it were going to pound right through my rib," but he continued the thirty-five-minute ride, feeling just a little sore the next day. After three months of daily commuting, his weight dropped twenty-five pounds, his heart rate dropped about 15 bpm, both blood pressure readings dropped 10 psi, and his cholesterol dropped 10 points to 190, though the LDL/HDL ratio improved significantly. "My blood concentration of triglycerides," he notes, "went from borderline risk to very good. All measurements held steady from then on. All ailments attributed to high stress went away." As of this writing, he has ridden his bike to work more than 700 times, using the bus or car only a few times during bad weather.

What began as a weight loss program has become a lifestyle. Gary jokes about what people consider bad weather. His daily bicycle commuting taught him there's no such thing as bad weather. "There is wet weather (hurricane remnants), cold (−15°F) weather, windy (45 mph) weather, overcast weather, and snowy weather but none of it is 'bad' to me anymore."

Gary drastically changed not only his health but also his perception. Weather that once was not fit for man or beast is now fit for him and he's fit for it. Cycling regularly invites or demands a context. And cycling offers a more compelling context than comparable sports. You can commute to work, ride with your family and clubs, cycle for a charity such as MS, go on-road or off-road, take your bike on vacation, at home or abroad, climb mountains or pound the pavement, ride centuries, race in citizens events or amateur and professional events, and so on. Wherever you are on the continuum of health, cycling will meet you there as it met Joe Green of Maxwell, Iowa, who went from being a 135-pound runner on a 6′ 1″ frame to a weight that fluctuated between 220 and 235 pounds, all in the course of a few years. A disk problem eliminated running as his preferred exercise so he went down that old familiar road and purchased a used Raleigh at his local bike shop, then upgraded to a Trek. Though he enjoyed cycling, he found that the weight did not melt from his frame and his doctor put him on blood pressure medication, advising him to lose 30 pounds. Joe was concerned and had good reason. His grandfather had died at age fifty-three and his brother at thirty-nine. Both parents take medication to control blood pressure.

The spirit was willing but the flesh weak. Gary returned to school and his weight shot up to 232 pounds. His life threatened, he decided to act. This time, however, he would not only ride the bike as often as possible "but also cut out junk food and really keep track of what I ate. No more doughnuts, regular soda, or chips. I cut down drastically on fried food (a passion of mine)."

He rode as much as possible and found the weight came off easily. He lost 35 pounds and could dispense with blood pressure medication. His back aches only when he doesn't ride, and the pain recurs occasionally as a prick of conscience. A 10–20-mile ride takes care of his back. Yes, he purchased a new Trek. Yes, his family thinks he's obsessed. Yes, he is riding centuries. And yes, cycling has become a lifestyle.

The old paradigm invokes itself. You look in the mirror and resolve to do something about your weight. Drag the bike out of the basement and pedal around the neighborhood. You get better and so does the bike. Where in the past you couldn't imagine walking a few blocks, you can now dream about cycling long distances. You find a challenge, perhaps a local century or metric century. Train for it. The weight drops. Your diet has changed. You enjoy life and your family more. Instead of watching television, you go for a bike ride.

I cannot do justice to the great emotional, physical, and spiritual struggles these people have undergone in losing weight and changing their lives. If cycling were a friend, it would be patient, responsive, and long-suffering. The bicycle is ready when you are.

Jim Williford of St. Petersburg, Florida, successfully battled alcohol only to have another demon waiting: his condition. Two years ago he weighed 256 pounds, had a 45-inch waist, and a 17.5 neck size. He tried running but his knees couldn't tolerate the pounding. He had a department store road bike but his stomach was so large he couldn't lean over enough to ride comfortably. So he purchased a Trek hybrid. At first he could ride only a few hundred yards without coasting but found conditioning came very quickly. He purchased a cycle computer and increased his mileage, average 11 mph.

In addition to exercise, he changed his diet, cutting out all fats and eating primarily fruits and vegetables. He remembers one afternoon when he "ate five or six bananas, four apples, a bunch of grapes, a couple of pears, and a few slices of bread" and was still hungry. Only a hot dog could satisfy him. Yet he persevered, mastering a food addiction and losing his craving for fat.

Jim joined a bike club, which helped him increase his speed to 12–15 mph, purchased clipless pedals, and put road tires on his bike. He got even faster and increased the duration, intensity, and frequency of his training. An average week was 250 miles. In his words, "I simply placed a priority on riding and it become the first thing I did after I got home from work. I also began cross-training at a local country and western dance club. Let me tell you, a night of line dancing rivals a hundred-mile race in exercise. The pounds began to fall away. I consistently lost four pounds per week for three months straight. When getting in shape through running, I would always hold weight for a few weeks, then plummet to a plateau and then hold for a few weeks until another plateau. With bicycling, I simply lost four pounds per week consistently."

After a year, his weight is down to 208 (a loss of 48 pounds), his waist is 38, and his neck 16. His resting pulse is 48 bpm. Jim rode 260 miles across Florida in a little under 11 hours, averaging 18 mph. He does training rides at 22 mph and has seen 35 mph on his cycle computer. Because he deserved it, Jim purchased a new, lighter bike with Italian components.

Jim Williford made a complete lifestyle change and has added to his life expectancy. He exudes happiness and pride. Jim exalts in putting his head down and cycling into the Florida wind.

Within this story is a life in turmoil and change. Perhaps a book in itself. To recover from the twin addictions of alcohol and fatty foods is a genuine accomplishment. To do so in a way that adds meaning and significance to life is a blessing. Jim went from tooling around the neighborhood at 11 mph to leading his Florida pack at 22 mph. Speed begets speed, mileage begets mileage. Yet as important as these accomplishments is the psychological change that allows one to more fully embrace life and take on greater challenges. One reason for this, I believe, is that with bicycling one also inherits a kind of psychology. The bike is light, strong, and delicately drawn with speed written all over it. As you have seen, few people who have tasted cycling can be happy with a department store bike because it's not light, fast, or responsive enough. Because the bike is mobility, it plays to our fantasies and dreams. And who doesn't dream of going fast, of being a wisp in the wind. Of the thousands of recreational cyclists I have interviewed, few don't warmly remember childhood cycling experiences and often invoke that memory when they climb aboard the bike as an adult. The claim that you never forget to ride a bike is true. Yet that statement holds for most of us more than the physics of balance. We hold memories of youth particularly dear because they are innocent and simple. The bike by its very nature is simple and that is part of its appeal. The bicycle is the most efficient machine ever invented for converting muscle energy into mechanical energy. I believe somehow the body knows this and cooperates. If you never forget how to ride a bike, the bike never forgets how to carry you. And carry you it does.

In collecting stories for this book, I've been struck by the care with which people monitor their health after deciding to start a weight loss cycling program. Two years ago Charles R. Haynsworth III, of Danville, Virginia, was 298 pounds on a 6' 4" frame. His cholesterol was 230, with the LDL cholesterol too high and the HDL too low. He started walking for exercise, and within a month he could cover 3 miles in under 36 minutes. However, his knees hurt so much he had to take twelve Motrin tablets each day to ease the pain.

He began cycling and after a season is in the best shape of his life. His weight is down to 216, cholesterol down to 150, and his body fat down to 15.5% from almost 30%. His chronic knee pain has disappeared since he started cycling. He eats better, cycles faster, and enjoys life more. Haynsworth watched his health with the eye of a physician. And his doctor must be well pleased.

I have athlete friends who claim that, because they exercise regularly, they can eat anything they want, which seems to be true for some. That is, as long as what they want is high is carbohydrates. One friend consumes a large bag of potato chips after a long bike ride and wonders why he doesn't lose weight. It's axiomatic that if you are overweight and want to lose weight through cycling, you'll have to pay close attention to your diet. To be sure cycling, done in the way described in this book, is a great calorie burner. If you are cycling in the right gear at a desirable cadence within your target heart zone, you will lose weight and get fitter. And as you get fit, your health will improve. Let's look at the numbers, using Jim Williford as an example. When he got in shape, Jim was pedaling at a brisk 22 mph. For the sake of convenience, we'll put his weight at 200 pounds. At that weight and speed he'll burn approximately 21.5 calories a minute, or almost 1,300 calories an hour. That is, if all things are equal and they never are. You have to take into consideration terrain, wind, and riding conditions. Keep in mind that few recreational cyclists move at that pace nonstop for an hour so you should adjust the numbers to fit your actual riding style and pace. Obviously, heavier cyclists will burn more calories at the same speed than lighter cyclists. For example, I'm 160 pounds and would burn 220 fewer calories an hour than Jim. That is, if I could keep up with him. Again, these numbers reflect an ideal picture. The wind hasn't started to blow or the hills to grow.

James Hagberg, Ph.D., and his colleagues at the University of Florida have conducted road studies to determine caloric expenditures under varying conditions and have developed various formulas to that end. If you ride hills you'll expend more calories than during a flat ride. In terms of calorie expenditure, ascents and descents almost balance each other out. As noted earlier, some riders cycle into the wind for training and that regimen burns extra calories, especially if the head wind is strong. However, you'll likely give up this gain if you have a tail wind on the ride home.

Riding position at speeds above 15 mph can also affect calorie burn. When riding on the drops, you'll expend fewer calories than if your hands are on the bars or brake hoods. If you are using panniers, you will increase slightly your caloric expenditure. If you are drafting another rider at 16 mph, the number of calories you burn will be less. However, most cyclists take turns drafting, and after 2–3 hours of hard riding, you might not be interested in counting. You'll feel the burn in your legs. Conversely, when mountain biking over tough terrain, throw all the numbers out the window. One hour on the mountain bike could be worth two on the road.

We can determine a baseline for calorie expenditure. But these numbers represent ideals, not always consistent with cycling in the real world, where we often loaf, tuck in behind another rider, coast downhills or freewheel on the flats, and let the wind blow us home after a hard ride. My general rule of thumb is that you probably burn fewer calories than an ideal baseline chart would suggest, sometimes as much as 20–30 percent less. But rather than calculating every variable, I suggest you underestimate the number of calories you burn. Balance your training accordingly. On the days you train primarily in the hills, figure you are closer to the ideal baseline numbers than when you go out for an easy spin. No cheating on your diet that night. On days you ride into a head wind but catch a tail wind home, figure it's a wash. Remember this research and these numbers were developed for road cyclists. If you ride a mountain bike on a rugged single track, you'll likely not be able to hold the speed you can on the road but could still burn an equal number of calories because of the intensity of the workout and the involvement of the upper body. I should add that there are certain heart rate monitors on the market that compute calories burned during a ride but they don't take into consideration terrain, wind, and other pertinent factors.

The calorie game is actually quite simple. Figure there are 3,500 calories in a pound. To determine your calorie need, multiply your weight by 15. Then, in round numbers, add 9 calories for every minute of cycling you do. At 160 pounds my body requires 2,400 calories a day. I cycled two hours today at an average speed of 16 mph. The ideal baseline suggests I expended 9.8 calories per minute cycling or about 1,176 calories. I was in rolling hills with a tail wind on the way out and a head wind on the way back. I felt strong and worked at about 70 percent of my maximum heart rate (this is early season). I didn't use the big chainring and tended to stay in the low and middle gears. So the number is probably fairly accurate. In all, I expended 3,576 calories today, and since I didn't eat that much, say 2,500 calories, I might have "lost" a fraction of a pound. This kind of analysis is good enough for me and perhaps for you. I'm not a slave to the last round number and the last granola bar consumed. I do collect the numbers, but always visit the mirror for confirmation. I always assume I have burned fewer calories than the charts show.

Calorie requirements are a half-stop on the way to the equally important subject of complex carbohydrates, which we know as pasta and potatoes. When you eat pasta, it's broken down into blood glucose, which ultimately serves as fuel for your ride. To make progress with a weight loss program, you'll want 65 percent of your total diet to be made up of carbohydrates. That means I'd need 1,460 calories from complex carbohydrates, or about 365 grams (there are 4 calories to a gram of carbohydrates).

No discussion of weight loss is complete without mentioning fat, both body and dietary. Body fat, referring to the percentage of total body weight that is composed of fat, is best measured by skin calipers or an underwater displacement test. Most YMCAs, gyms, and sports medicine labs will be able to assist. The "pinch test," though not necessarily reliable, can be revealing. So can a look in the naked mirror. Men and women bike racers usually have 7% and 14% of body fat, respectively. The average American male carries about 20% body fat, the average female 28%. As a recreational cyclist, you'll likely want to be around 10–15% if you are male and 14–20% if female. But these are rough ranges that will depend on your body type. I'd recommend you shoot for the low end of the range. I know cyclists who remain strong and fresh at 5% body fat but there is evidence if you get too low you will become fatigued. Women should be careful getting below 12% because they could stop menstruating. I've heard exercise physiologists claim that cyclists carry enough fat to enable them to do 300 miles without a break, so most of us are well equipped in the fat zone. Moreover, since large amounts of oxygen are required to convert fat to energy, you can burn only when sufficient air is available, up to 50–60% of maximum heart rate. You tend to burn more fat when you increase your training duration, frequency, and intensity. Your body will turn to fat stores for energy when you burn more calories than you consume. Some racers actually believe you can teach your body to burn fat into the higher target zones, say up to 80% of maximum. One way is to do long, easy rides, forcing the body to use the fat supply. Another way is to go on a ride without breakfast and don't eat for an hour or more. Fat energy will kick in after the body depletes its glycogen or stored carbohydrates.

One of the best ways to reduce body fat is to cut down on dietary fat. In this case you are what you eat. The average American gets about 38–40% of his or her diet from fat. That's a whopping percentage. Ironically, it's not always fast food that is the major offender. Nutritionists estimate that up to two-thirds of dietary fat comes not from burgers but from oils, dairy products, nuts, pastries, and snacks. Those are the items to watch. Instead of being a calorie counter, be a fat watcher, because it's dietary fat that is most often converted to body fat. Almost all the cyclists mentioned in this chapter attacked fat as aggressively as they attacked the hills and watched their body fat plummet with their dietary fat intake. That is axiomatic. Ideally, you want 20–25% of your calories to be from fat, with no more than 10% coming from saturated fats found in animal products. The rest should come from unsaturated fats such as oils, nuts, and the like. If you are a 120-pound woman, your calorie intake should be 1,400 with a fat intake of 39 grams, the way it is listed on nutritional charts on foods. Jim Williford can consume 78 grams of fat on a total diet of 2,800 calories. I can consume 2,200 calories and 61 grams of fat. Each gram of fat equals 9 calories. So 9 calories multiplied by 61 equals 549 calories, which represents about 25% of my total daily calorie intake. As a rule of thumb, most people can manage on about 40 grams of dietary fat a day. I try to be closer to that number than the 61. You or someone in the household must become a label reader. Try to avoid foods that contain more than 20 grams a serving as that would be 50% of the daily fat requirement for most people. Or looking at this another way, avoid foods that contain more than 3–4 grams of fat for each 100-calorie serving.

Keeping a close eye on your fat intake and cycling 3–4 times a week at least 40 minutes each time should ensure that you will lose 2 pounds a week, perhaps more. With training, the body can store significantly more glycogen, which will make a difference on your long, fat-depleting miles. As you have seen, one cyclist reported consistently losing 4 pounds a week for up to 3 months, which is more likely to occur if you have a lot to lose. But be realistic. Don't expect too much, too fast. By all means keep a food diary for a week and look for patterns. Do you binge on weekends, throwing the week's gains out the window? Do you consume junk food after a hard ride, feeling that's the reward for hard work? Do you eat one big meal a day rather than spreading out the calories?

After a point, a weight loss regimen is common sense. If you want to lose weight, you'll likely have to give up or cut down on nuts, chips, cheese, ice cream, cookies, peanut butter, and the like. The key is to replace these foods with low-fat alternatives. I offer a seven-day menu in the appendixes that is designed to satisfy your appetite yet encourage sensible weight loss.

As you increase your mileage, an inevitable part of your program, be sensitive to food intake. Don't starve yourself to get the weight off quicker. Your performance will suffer. If you ride an hour a day, at least 60% of your total calories should come from complex carbohydrates (beans, cereals, grains, etc.); 70% if you ride more than two hours.

In the next chapter, I'll be discussing in more detail on-bike nutrition. In closing this chapter, I want to reiterate a few simple rules of thumb: If you ride regularly and reduce your fat intake, you will lose weight. Though you may lose more, a sensible weight loss program will mean a loss of 2 pounds a week. As we saw from Joe Green's experience cited in this chapter, you can ride a bike and still not lose weight. Unless you are doing very heavy mileage, you won't lose weight without modifying your diet as needed. Or if you do, it's not likely to be permanent.

A cycling weight loss program is ideal for old and young, man or woman, athlete or physically impaired. After all the calories are counted and grams consumed, it's a matter of getting on the bike, which is sometimes a matter of life and death. Consider James Lazado of Grindstone, Pennsylvania, who at age forty-four weighed 232 pounds at a height of 5′ 7″. He thought he was having a heart attack. Not so, said his doctor. It was his poor condition and bad eating habits. He bought an exercise bike, refurbished his road bike, and purchased a mountain bike, and in six months he reduced his weight to 165 pounds through regular cycling and improved eating habits. He now cycles more than 6,000 miles a year.

You can too.

POWER EATING

Ernest Hemingway loved sports and used to write about hunting, deep-sea fishing, and bullfighting. Who can forget the artistry of the bullfight scenes in *The Sun Also Rises*? Hemingway reveled in the moments when hunter and hunted became one, bestowing on each a kind of majesty. Throughout his career he saluted moments of grace under pressure and chased that demon personally through his tumultuous life. He liked the clean lines of the bullfight, the boxing ring, or the bike race. And these moments in sport and life became compressed in the language of his novels and short stories. His sentences are short in length, active in voice, and largely free of decoration. He eschewed abstract words such as "honor" and "courage" and celebrated concrete place names that still had meaning and character.

I don't know why I think of Hemingway when I think of the bicycle. Perhaps it's the clean lines, the simple geometry, the elegance. Hemingway described the moment in which the matador is one with the bull, before the *coup de grâce*. The scene makes a clean and perfect line. The bicycle offers a similar prospect to the serious rider. Think about it. When you are aboard a bike, your position is defined in relation to the geometry of the bike. Knee at a certain angle to the crank, nose over the stem and dissecting the front hub, back at an angle to the top tube. Being one with the bike is far from a cliché uttered by those in the saddle too long. Being one with the bike is certainly about fit but it's also about feel and aesthetics. With feet in clipless pedals, you are closer to the mechanics of power and therefore

165

are more powerful. Sitting over the rear wheel as you drop down a mountain at 35 mph makes you part of the bike's geometry and center of gravity. Wearing cycling gloves, shorts, shoes, helmet, and jersey is only slightly about fashion. Wearing this gear is mainly about aesthetics and aerodynamics. You want to go fast and look fast too. Whether you're on the road or single track, you want to look the part because you are playing a kind of synecdoche, a part for the whole. And the whole is speed, weightlessness, and balancing on air.

Watch a professional racer or a good amateur and the movements on the bike are fluid and smart, whether shifting into a higher gear or reaching for the water bottle. Clean lines all over again. Watch the way he or she gets out of the saddle, preparing to climb. The movement is that of a cat, water flowing uphill. This cat is not on a rocking horse but on a frame that barely twitches under enormous muscle power. One reason we like to watch world champions Lance Armstrong, Ned Overend, and Juli Furtado is that we want to look like them and then perhaps ride like them. And looking good on a bike is not about vanity. If your body makes the clean lines and angles with road and bike, you will likely cycle more efficiently and get better, faster. If you understand the gearing and make the frequent incremental shifts to match your fitness and the terrain, you are celebrating the bicycle. If you "kiss" the brakes rather than gripping them like a final handshake, you are riding clean and sure. And if you give the same care and attention to your body that you give to the bike, you are truly one with the machine.

THE RIGHT NUTRIENTS

Looking good on a bike means feeling good and that means having the right nutrients in the system when needed. Cycling is the rare activity that demands you consume food while you are actually doing it. What you eat on the bike is as important as what you eat at home. Actually, these are complementary activities—one should anticipate the other. The power you bring to cycling comes from the training you do and the food you eat. The weight you lose while cycling will depend heavily on what you eat both on and off the bike. It was not that long ago that I remember cyclists stopping for three or four beers and a large pizza during a bike tour lunch break. Another cyclist who actually rode across the country trained on a diet heavy with beer. He said it gave him energy and somehow he completed the ride in decent time. Consider him the exception. Drinking beer before, during, or too soon after a ride is not in the interest of your health and nutrition. Come to think of it, my story must be at least ten years old. Even the most casual cyclists these days seem to know that what you put into your system significantly affects your power output. You even see this at the major races where the content of the feed bag, which is passed to racers at key points along the race route, has changed mightily. The feed bag, or "musette" (small bag), used to be full of rolls stuffed with a variety of meats and cheeses which were heavy, very high in fat content, difficult to digest, and tended to leave riders short on energy long before they reached the finish line. Giving racers solid food high in protein seemed the right thing to do. After all, they were working hard and needed something that stuck to their ribs, which is precisely the same sentiment that prompted my mother to give my father eggs, bacon, and sausage for breakfast every morning. (Thank goodness I was stuck with the lowly oatmeal.) We now know that pork rolls and ham sandwiches can sit in the stomach for 3–4 hours and don't contribute much in the way of energy. The blood is rushing to the stomach to aid digestion rather than rushing to the legs, which are screaming for help. Now when riders are passed the musette, it will likely contain fruit or an energy bar. Even today, Tour de France riders are getting more of their carbohydrate fuel from liquid sources because it supplies energy within minutes in the form the body needs. Moreover, a lot of the commercial (and homemade) energy drinks are 10 percent carbohydrates and that gives a quick boost to a racer. So does Coca-Cola, which is used in diluted form by many racers.

A hundred years ago racers generally competed without any particular concern about food. When many collapsed before the finish line, thought was given to on-bike nutrition but few advances were made until the last two decades. I can still remember taking sandwiches on long rides. We now know that the body can store enough carbohydrates, in the form of glycogen, for short rides. Therefore, if you commute to work or go for short rides in the neighborhood, nutrition is something that you can get at home. However, if you take longer rides, your glycogen stores will be depleted and will have to be refilled. If not, you'll feel weak, light-headed, and perhaps dizzy. I affectionately called this condition the "bonk" the few times I reached it when running marathons, though I've experienced it only once while cycling. I was riding across Pennsylvania at the end of a 100-mile day deep in the mountains and I couldn't turn the pedals anymore. I fell over and had to rest and eat before I could continue. I later learned that my liver glycogen stores were depleted. My companion and I had pushed on without stopping for lunch, and I paid the price. Since that time, whenever I have felt weary and lethargic on a bike I tend to respond before my condition worsens. Please keep in mind that a lot of so-called serious cyclists "bonk," many with food in their pockets and energy replacement drinks in their packets. Be vigilant.

ANTICIPATE FATIGUE

If I'm going out for an hour or more, I usually take something to eat, if only a banana. And I always take a water bottle. Every cyclist knows that you drink before you're thirsty and eat before you're hungry. That's another mantra you should attach to your handlebars. I drink from my water bottle every 10–20 minutes, depending on the weather. But even in the cold weather you can dehydrate. I'm writing this in February, and I went out for a 2-hour ride the other day and came back short on water—I had taken one bottle rather than two. A good rule of thumb is to take along a 20-ounce water bottle for every hour of cycling. Likewise start nibbling on fruit or an energy bar after you've been on the road more than an hour. You'll certainly want to replicate on the bike the high carbohydrate meals you eat at home. Candy bars are a handy item to put in your jersey pocket, but try to avoid them because they are high in fat, which is an ineffective fuel source. So I can be virtuous and satisfied at the same time, I have been known to combine a banana and a Baby Ruth. But I always ride better after the banana.

Australian researchers have developed a glycemic index to rate foods high in glycogen. Cyclists who had consumed foods high on the glycemic index (corn flakes, raisins, whole wheat, potatoes, sports drinks, carrots, etc.) had less glucose in their blood after riding 100 minutes on a stationary bike than cyclists who had consumed food low on the glycemic index (apple, dates, figs, yogurt). This finding means or could mean that the low-index cyclists would have been able to go longer and faster. However, we store glucose in our muscles as glycogen and have enough for only about two hours of effort, so you would be advised to replenish your glycogen stores with a shot of a high-indexing sports drink or a banana, which falls in the middle of the index. Likewise these same foods have been found to be ideal for replacing carbohydrate stores after a ride.

Keep in mind that much of this advice will be useful after you are well into your training program. In season, I regularly cycle 34 miles round trip to work. Before I leave, I might have toast and a banana or nothing, and for that amount of time in the saddle, it makes little difference. When I get to work, I'll eat oatmeal or cereal, but not as much as I might if I hadn't cycled. We know cycling does suppress the appetite slightly. But if I'm going out on a 50-mile training ride, I'll try to eat fruit and grain an hour or two before the ride. If not, I'll snack on an energy bar of some kind. I know that, once the ride starts, I'll go easy for the first half hour. By then I figure the glucose is in my bloodstream and feeding the muscles. I also know the effect of the breakfast will wear off after a little more than an hour, so before that time, I have eaten a banana or I'm chewing on an energy bar. If not, I'll be taking some energy drink. One rule of thumb suggests you should consume 60–100 grams of carbohydrates for every hour on the bike. That's 240–400 calories. Most cyclists know that fatigue comes like an unwelcome guest at mile 30–36, a little over the two-hour riding mark for many cyclists in training. Conventional wisdom suggests you should anticipate fatigue by at least half an hour, and nibbling constantly but strategically is one way to do this. By the time you get within 30 minutes of home, rely on energy drinks. And once home, replenish your carbohydrate supplies. For example, at 160 pounds I would probably need to consume about 120 grams of carbohydrates or 480 calories within two hours for optimal utilization. Most cyclists find that energy drinks are the best and quickest way to refuel. Not only will you recover more quickly from the ride, but you'll also be better prepared, nutritionally speaking, for riding the next day.

In competitive racing circles I hear talk about the need for more protein. Coaches frequently start their riders with a breakfast of eggs and bacon rather than pancakes, the traditional morning meal for the recreational cyclist. One coach says, "I hate pancakes. I believe in protein for longevity on the bike. This means ham and eggs." Though many competitive cyclists likely need more protein than they're getting, a condition that can cause fatigue, this has little application for most recreational cyclists, who need primarily carbohydrates and probably get enough incidental protein anyway. Protein simply can't match carbohydrates for delivering energy when needed. If you consume an energy bar or part of one at 8 A.M., the food is converted to glucose by about 8:30 A.M. and shortly afterward finds its way into your muscles, ready for use. A high-fat product might be 8 hours behind and will not be as effective when it is converted for use by the muscles.

A PROFESSIONAL'S DIET

Here is a sample one-day diet for Tour de France racer Ron Kiefel, who can burn up to 10,000 calories in a day.

Breakfast, normally eaten 3 hours before the start of a race (1,833 calories, consisting of 62% carbohydrates, 24% fat, 14% protein): Cereal, muesli, Froot Loops, or a combination with soy milk. Coffee or chocolate to drink. A two-egg omelet with cheese or ham or two fried eggs for protein. Pasta or rice without topping for carbohydrates. Perhaps some bread and jam or a croissant with jam. A bottle of water.

Before the race: A piece of fruit.

During the race (3,632 calories—97% carbohydrates, 2% protein, 1% fat): Two muesli bars, stored in his jersey pocket, to be eaten within the first 40 miles or less than 2 hours. At the two feed zones, each rider has a choice of 3–4 muesli bars, a PowerBar, a small can of Coke, two water bottles (one filled with a carbohydrate drink), and two containers of a liquid glucose solution. During a typical race Ron consumes ten bottles of liquid.

After the race (919 calories—78% carbohydrates, 12% protein, 9% fat): A quart of water immediately. Within an hour a bowl of muesli or a sandwich to start replenishing carbohydrates.

Dinner (2,304 calories—44% carbohydrates, 35% fat, 18% protein): Pasta without sauce. Salad. Fish, chicken, or steak. Potatoes and cooked vegetables. Sometimes a glass of wine. Cheese, yogurt, or a fruit tart for dessert.

Of the nearly 9,000 calories the racer consumes, 73% are carbohydrate, 16% fat, and 10% protein, not a bad model to emulate in principle. (On the other hand, I've seen studies that indicate some Tour riders eat a diet as high as 39% fat.) Note that Ron's breakfast is far heavier in protein than most fitness riders would require. During the race your on-bike diet and his should be similar in terms of where the calories come from. And he is very conscious about replenishing his carbohydrate stores after a race. After all he does this for a living. He'll race another 6–7 hours the next day, a stage in the almost month-long, 2,000-mile journey called the Tour de France.

Tour de France riders have coaches, trainers, and nutritionists who help them select their daily bread. Unfortunately, we are not so lucky and have to rely on our wits and whatever advice we pick up along the way. By and large, I've found cyclists ahead of the general population when it comes to knowledge about nutrition. Some of this information has come the hard way, such as after experiencing the deadly "bonk" and pulling in last on a century ride, not because of poor fitness, but owing to poor nutrition. My suggestion is that after you take all this diverse (and sometimes conflicting) information into your head, experiment and choose a program that seems right for you. Too much has already been written about a preride meal. I've told you what I do and suggested some alternatives. Experiment on your training rides and go with the system that seems better.

I recall on a tour of Britain last year a friend who could eat two or three entrées. So surprised by his appetite, the waiter in an Indian restaurant in the Midlands almost refused to serve him. He simply didn't believe my friend could eat all that food. We tried to explain that we had ridden 100 miles and had done so for the last four days, and that my friend was hungry. My friend got the food, ate everything, and was ready for another PowerBar in an hour.

If you race or train hard and long, it's sometimes difficult to consume enough calories, especially when you are away from food sources, such as in the Scottish Highlands early Sunday morning. But even when you work a 40-hour week, ride 150–200 miles, and keep up with the myriad responsibilities of a family, it's hard to consume enough "benevolent" calories—and what often follows is the rush to junk food. One solution is to eat four or five small meals a day rather than the traditional Big Three. Research has shown you can actually lose weight this way.

Cyclists love to eat. Just stop at a restaurant or food stop along an organized tour route to witness the acres of bananas and baloney sandwiches. The joy of eating naturally flows from the joy of cycling. However, on numerous occasions I've seen cyclists cancel out their on-bike gains, including weight loss, achieved during a ride by what they eat along the way, at a food stop or at an end-of-the-ride binge. Here are some tips to keep you in shape and losing weight even when you're on the bike.

COMMERCIAL ENERGY PRODUCTS

I've already confessed my sin about Baby Ruth, which is well known among my friends, who regularly tempt me when we stop at convenience stores for something edible. I'm getting better, said the addict. I haven't had one in a year and I never carry them with me. My on-bike, nutritious snack of choice is the energy bar, which is so reliable I used to take large quantities to Russia when I first visited that country six years ago (not to sell; to eat). Trouble is the energy bar business is no longer a cottage industry but big business. Today, a decade after PowerBar popularized the market, there are nearly thirty rivals out there. I've tasted and used most on a bike, testing for taste, digestion, and ease of opening. I've read the labels, looking for nutritional content as grams of fat and the percentage of complex carbohydrates. Most fitness cyclists want a high-carbohydrate low-fat energy bar that tastes good, is easy to open, digests well, and doesn't contain too many calories. PowerBar, Performance, Exceed, PurePower, and Clif Bar generally satisfy these requirements. The nutritional content is on the wrapper, but taste is very personal. Though PowerBar has made some improvements, I can't stand the chocolate flavor. Yet a friend consumes this chocolate bar as if it were caviar. At times I've had difficulty opening most energy bar wrappers but that's because my hands are greasy from repairing a chain, it's raining, or my fingers are simply too cold. (Hint: Break the seal before leaving the house.)

Like energy drinks, energy bars proliferate and can be found right alongside that Baby Ruth on candy counters. Be careful. Some bars such as Kellogg's Nutri-Grain, Meal on the Go, and Balance have a high fat content. In fairness, the last is advertised as a meal replacement and is also high in protein. Whatever the advertisement says, you want most of your on-bike nutrition to come from carbohydrates that are readily available to the muscles. You can find more enjoyable ways to consume protein.

If there has been a proliferation of commercial energy bars, there's been an accompanying surge in the number of energy drinks and concentrated carbohydrate drinks coming to the market. So successful have they been that most fitness and performance cyclists use one kind or another. Energy drinks contain up to 10% carbohydrates, which fuel the muscles and counter dehydration. Some drinks contain traces of electrolytes, which can be lost during hard training. The recommended energy drinks contain glucose rather than fructose because the former delivers more carbohydrates. Gatorade dominates the market, though Exceed and ERG are popular with cyclists. I regularly use Gatorade on my long training rides, often diluting it with half-part water. Again, this is a personal preference rather than body chemistry talking. I have difficulty consuming a lot of an energy drink, especially on an empty stomach. On overnight trips I will usually take a powdered energy drink to mix in my water bottle each morning.

Concentrated carbo drinks have a higher percentage of carbohydrates than energy drinks, usually around 20%. Research has shown that solutions over 12% carbohydrates don't empty out of the stomach quickly and can cause nausea. For that reason a lot of these products are best suited for before- or after-ride consumption. Long-distance and ultramarathon cyclists, such as those who compete in the Race Across America, swear by these concentrated liquids and have used them successfully under strenuous conditions. As with other products, you should experiment with Ultra Energy, Carboloader, Gatorlode, and other energy drinks to see how your system responds. If they are too hard on your stomach during a ride, consider using them as a preride meal.

With more and more fruit juices showing up in vending machines, you are more likely these days to have more drinks to choose from. From research done on long-distance cyclists, we know those consuming glucose did better than those using sucrose and fructose, in that order. Still, fruit juices can provide a change of pace and still fuel your muscles. Libby's has a line of juices that is fairly high in carbohydrates and potassium, especially the Banana Nectar. Be careful of orange juices and those containing a lot of corn syrup, which is largely sucrose. Again, experiment on your training rides.

Obviously, we can't carry all the food needed for long tours in our bike jersey pocket and are often obliged to stop at convenience stores. Sometimes I think I'm the reason store personnel put chips, nuts, and candy next to the store entrance. I've actually given up nuts, chips, and candy but that wasn't always the case. The spirit was willing but my flesh was weak. (I feel an explanation is in order. I used to indulge in these items on multiday trips, but I now know I was bad. *Mea culpa.*) Eat several ounces of chips and you consume more than 300 calories, almost 60% from fat. Nuts are worse. In this aisle, pretzels are the better bet. Cookies, candy bars, and cakes contribute little to your cycling performance but a lot to your waist. Avoid them like the plague. Instead find the fruit counter and eat a banana, which costs a fraction of a sports drink, carbo drink, or energy bar but has an equivalent number of carbohydrates (30 grams) and fewer calories. For a cyclist, this is a best buy because it's portable, cheap, easy to digest, and nutritious. I rarely leave home, even on a short ride, without a few sticking out of my jersey pocket.

On long trips, cyclists are sometimes forced to stop at a fast-food restaurant, usually out of desperation, really; I've been there. My best advice is to pass on the 600-calorie Big Mac and get a chicken sandwich without the junk. Same with pizza. If you must indulge, go with the pizza that has the most dough or crust. Forget the meat topping and go with as little cheese as possible. Some places such as Domino's actually accept low-fat cheese orders. Or ask them to hold the extra cheese. Few restaurant pizzas come with less than 30% fat. So if you do indulge, take that into consideration.

Few large group rides don't end with a pasta meal. Good reason. Pasta is a profile of a fairly healthy diet as it consists of 70% carbohydrate, 10% protein, and 20% fat. No wonder it's the ideal meal before or after a long ride. More exotic pastas, including spinach and beet, contain significantly greater amounts of fat and cholesterol. But the real problem with pasta is what we put on it. Heavy cream, butter, and cheese sauces can significantly increase both the fat content and the calories in pasta, thus largely negating the health effects. A serving of Alfredo can be well over 1,000 calories and 43 grams of fat, the daily fat requirement for a lot of Americans.

Try to reduce fat content of sauces by using olive oil. Be wary of stuffed pastas because they can contain up to 30–40% fat. And eliminate macaroni and cheese because its calorie and fat content are off the chart compared to its nutritional value.

To develop your clean power line while cycling, you'll naturally come to power foods. You cannot fill your stomach with junk food, empty calories, and simple carbohydrates and lose weight while developing your prowess as a cyclist. You have noticed that one theme repeated again and again in this book is what I call the "inevitable bike upgrade." People customarily begin a cycling program with what's at hand, usually a reliable, heavy department store bike parked in the basement. With success, the bike becomes too heavy, cumbersome, not a projection of the user's dreams and imagination. A better bike enters the house. Leaner, cleaner-looking, inviting the cyclist to be just that. A beautifully finished titanium bike is no more majestic than you, who have come back to life through cycling. You shine as much, look as good, are just as precious. The woman who named her bike Vishnu, the preserver god, is a goddess herself because she carved something beautiful from her old shape. She reinvented herself. Better bike, better cycling, better body, and better life all commingle, and to put all that under a weight loss banner does their majesty a disservice. The whole is greater than the sum of its parts. By now you know weight loss is a goal, the bike the vehicle, the long ride your strategic plan. But success in this venue implodes and grows new nerve endings, permitting you to take life in different ways. All these themes are clustered around the weight loss compass. Whichever way you go is the right way.

I've talked to enough cyclists to know that, when you take up cycling, the body, mind, and spirit all become engaged. Taste buds change. The bicycle civilizes and simplifies. The bicycle is a very basic mechanism, primitive in its elegance. By riding regularly, we become simpler in our wants. We eat lower on the food chain. Our perspective changes. We eschew fat the same way we do a heavy bike or a derailleur that shifts like old machinery. We know that food that does not quicken us is dead. That is not a political statement; rather, a poetic one. Bruce Randall of Springfield, Massachusetts, became a vegetarian for the practical reason that meat-centered meals weighed him down with heavy digestion and hurt his cycling, as if his center of gravity were thrown off.

Cycling, especially for weight loss, is about process. The bike moves under your power. Your muscles find the glycogen and convert it to muscular energy that turns the cranks. Your turning is in tune with the seasons, and when you hit the right note, make the right music, and pedal in the right cadence, you will lose weight, a little at a time, evenly because that's how the bike moves.

A recreational cyclist told me a long time ago, "if you don't eat right, you won't ride well." That's another axiom you can tape on your handlebars. Like your knowledge of gearing, you need to take your knowledge of nutrition inside, making it as much a part of you as new clothing. Sometimes you might have to wear it. Michael Tice, whom we have heard from before, does. He calls himself and his family "label-reading, fat-gram-counting, carbo-loading, sugar-scorning freaks. Nothing fried ever. No fast food ever. We make our own bread pizza crust and sauces. I force fluids all day, all week. Lots of juices and no alcohol. I don't feel this is anything special but our relatives think we are really weird. Of course, next to them we look adopted. We eat a lot of pasta and vegetables. On the bike I eat PowerBars and drink water or diluted Exceed. I take a couple of whole wheat rolls on a real long ride and drink a bottle every 30–45 minutes depending on the heat and the intensity of the ride. I never eat within 2 hours of a race."

I tend to think cycling is a mirror of the rest of our life. That is, how you live has a lot to do with how you cycle and how your body feels. John DeFayette of Schuyler Falls, New York, lost 30 pounds 6 years ago and has kept the weight off through cycling and a low-fat diet. He doesn't eat dessert or candy and is in better shape than he was fifteen years ago.

David Micales of Piscataway, New Jersey, had no weight loss plan. He ate smaller, more nutritious meals more frequently and he lost 20 pounds over a 5-year period. He does ride 6,000 miles a year and that might have something to do with the loss. But sometimes weight loss is an afterthought. Small adjustments can make a big difference over time. It's your body and schedule. Go easy, go fast. If, like Patrick Boylan of Burnsville, Minnesota, your body responds to the music of a gallon or more of water a day, do it. Figure out what keeps you moving. Listen to your body. Find your personal strategies that will help you lose weight and find, as he does, the "sweet spot" of cycling.

Time in the saddle does offer a certain reward. Michael K. Budak of Loman, Minnesota, has no real nutrition plan. He doesn't "figure up percentages of carbohydrates and fats. After all my years of racing, touring, and commuting, I know what works for me and what doesn't. Touring I average 100 miles a day and so pretty much cram down as much food as possible as many times a day as I can with whatever I can find. I am known as the 'Eating Machine' when on tour."

If this chapter is a screen, the last example might seem a camera out of focus. I don't mean to debunk the advice in this chapter; rather I'd like to remind you that we live in a world of doughnuts and Baby Ruths and, as you get better, you will have to ride through the market of cheap sugar tricks. Keep your sense of humor. Don't approach cycling as if it were a cult experience. It's play, and weight loss is that stuff that drips to the playground floor. Don't be too enamored of the technical. I've been fighting the impulse for years. Remember how it felt to ride a bike as a child. Think of the athletes who ride the Tour de France or those who cycle with one leg. Think of weight loss as a gift you give back to the bike for carrying you without shame. Think of the clean lines you make with your bike. And by all means keep moving.

SELF-CARE

Except for the time I caught someone's wheel, I've never been injured cycling. Just bruises and road and trail rash. I've been sore, tired, wiped out, short-tempered, angry, famished, depleted, bonked but never injured. I don't mean this as a boast. On the contrary, it's a statement of fact. I have run track and cross-country, have boxed, played fast-pitch softball, played football, baseball, and soccer and have experienced some kind of injury in the process. I love to run, race in 10Ks and marathons, but the event or the training usually leads to injury. I've had blisters on my butt but never bad enough to keep me out of the saddle. My back has ached and my neck has felt like a pylon receiving road shock, but never enough to derail me. As a matter of fact, the one time I went down hard, I immediately stopped at a convenience store, borrowed a package of frozen beans to treat my road rash, and climbed back on the bike. I paid later for that prideful act when the doctor picked pieces of the road out of my infected thigh and behind. I don't want to make light of the real dangers associated with cycling. You are often in traffic and that always presents a clear and present danger. But the more skilled you are with a bike, the less trouble you will have. The safest on-road cyclists are those who ride in traffic. Still, the traffic fear is a real one and encourages many people to buy mountain bikes and ride the single tracks.

When I refer to cycling as a soft exercise, some think the term refers to the ease of participating in the sport, and to a degree, that is true. But please don't mistake "ease" for "easy." Cycling is "soft" because it's easy on the body. You've seen numerous examples of people who cannot walk but can cycle. Anything I can offer pales in comparison to the courage and drive shown by the individuals who understand the profound psychological and spiritual ramifications of what scientists dryly call mobility. I am convinced that, beyond the rare accident for the skilled cyclist, one has to try to be injured as a cyclist. Usually the first to go is the knee, probably owing to pushing too big a gear too often in the season. I confess: it's happened to me. On a spring day with the wind just right, I have to fight the temptation of coaxing the chain onto the big ring. I recall a little more than a year ago on a ride from Land's End, England, to John o' Groat's, Scotland, I made the rookie mistake. It was August, so I had thousands of miles under my belt. Well-prepared, I felt invincible. The second day out, having been tired out by the surprisingly pricklish Cornwall hills, I rode too fast late in the day, gobbling up the villages during the last two hours of the trip, out of the saddle most of the time, and pushing too big a gear. I felt absolutely wonderful not because I had reached a bed and breakfast ten minutes ahead of my companion, but because I felt untouchable, liberated, and high. The next day, however, I felt a sharp pain in my knees and thigh muscles and had to slow down, spend more time off the bike, and push a decidedly smaller gear than I had wished. I was lucky that the knee pain left me on the fourth day. The bicycle is a beautiful machine, but I can't expect it to compensate for my stupidity.

No physiologist has ever fully explained to me the effect cycling has on the body's cellular level, or perhaps I just can't understand the talk. Cycling will tire you out but will likely never wear you out, at least not if you follow the training advice in this book. And a great chasm exists between these two states. No matter how well I train for a marathon, I can hardly walk the next day so I join the thousands of my sore brethren who descend stairs backward, thus easing the pain in a pantomime, a grotesque version of my mobility. Yet after I cycled almost 1,000 miles in 10 days with a 12-pound pack, I felt no ill effects with the exception of some saddle sores which, as I explain later in the chapter, I brought with me. On the contrary, I felt the beneficial effects of cycling through my body: in my weight, heart, muscles, and joints. I returned to London the next day and ran in Hyde Park. I felt I was running on circus stilts.

I want to reiterate that you usually have to work at being injured while cycling. In fact, cycling works wonders in the other direction. If you're injured in another sport, especially if it's a muscle injury, you can usually cycle. Not only will you be able to exercise but cycling will likely help you heal the injury. I'm writing this after a business trip that took me to Moscow, Munich, and Bath, England. Not much cycling that trip, except for a mountain bike excursion in Munich. Fortunately, the hotels in Munich and Bath had treadmills. Despite doing the requisite stretches, I pulled a calf muscle and could barely walk, let alone run. As soon as I got home, I climbed aboard my mountain bike and cycled with no pain. Cycling helped me recover.

My point is that cycling is inherently safe, injury-free, and almost protective of the body. People with severe leg injuries, balance problems, and nerve disorders can cycle and feel the pedals as if they were a part of them. On a bike you don't pound but float, moving over the most inhospitable terrain. You or a suspension system might absorb shock but you don't absorb injury. I feel sore after three winter road rides in a row for 35 miles each day over snow-ravaged surfaces. I had to take more punishment than I normally would but I'm sore, not injured. Furthermore, I got good practice jumping potholes, making a virtue out of necessity.

At the bottom of the pedal stroke you find air or gravity, not a harsh patch of pavement. There is no concussion. Your foot moves in a way so that neither your knee nor your hip is jarred. You can concentrate on your pedal motion, not foot placement, to reduce impact.

Biomechanics studies your relationship to the bicycle, the physics of what happens when man and machine come together. Frankly, I'm not interested in the forces that push this way and that, probably because I don't understand them well enough. One of the best books on this subject is *Bicycle Science*, by Professor David Gordon Wilson, a cycling enthusiast and colleague. I'm more interested in what the bicycle allows you to do, which, in a nutshell, is almost everything. The bicycle doesn't define you; it liberates you to do whatever you want.

The beginning of cycling self-care is to be on the right bike, a subject we have explored in great detail. You can probably ride almost anything, the body is so adaptable and the bike so forgiving, but you shouldn't. Pleasure does not come from sitting on a 2×4 at speed. Bicycle fit is the sine qua non of cycling. Everything flows from your proper biomechanical relationship with the bicycle. If I had to choose, I'd take a heavier bike rather than an ill-fitting one. A stem that is a few millimeters too long can stretch you out and make you most uncomfortable.

I haven't been a hawker of accessories in this book, but by now you know riding shorts, jersey, gloves, shoes, and helmet are a function of fit and comfort. You'll add to the cycling wardrobe as you get better, just like your brethren in these pages. Not only do these necessary accessories put you in better relationship with the wind, aerodynamically speaking, but they provide comfort and protection from the elements. Cycling shorts have a chamois lining that provides cushioning in one of the most sensitive areas of your body. Cycling shoes have a stiff shank which enables you to deliver power to the pedals without feeling as if you had the pedal cage surgically attached to the bottom of your foot. If you've tried to ride with running or fitness shoes, you'll know what I'm talking about. You last 10–15 miles, maybe, before your feet become numb. Padded gloves provide grip and shock absorption. The helmet speaks for itself.

NECESSARY ACCESSORIES

Let me echo those words: You should never climb aboard a bike for a ride around the block or across the nation without wearing a helmet. That is meant to be an unequivocal statement. Neither should your children be permitted to ride without a helmet. Long before helmets became fashionable, I was an ardent supporter of their use. I supported helmet use 15 years ago when the products were ugly, fit badly, and weighed so much they caused neck pain. And I said that in print. I've traveled the national television circuit encouraging everyone to wear this most necessary accessory. Fortunately the market has responded. Helmets come in more styles, shapes, and prices than most shops can handle. As I write this, there are at least a hundred models on the market competing for your attention. Average weight is about 9 ounces though some are as light as 6 or 7 ounces. Most are basically an expanded polystyrene shell with a thin plastic for covering. Others are made only of foam or hardshell. The "thin shell" is clearly the trend, with about 70 percent of the helmets on the market using this construction. Some come with a choice of helmet covers that you can use on different occasions. You can buy a helmet for around $40 or spend as much as $100 or more on a pumped-up, souped-up, high-tech model. For the high price you can wear what Olympic cyclists wear. The extra cost is usually in the design and do-dads. All helmets have a sticker on the inside stating they are approved by one testing laboratory or the other (usually Snell or ANSI). If the helmet doesn't have such a label, which means it's passed minimum drop and impact tests, don't buy it. Bell, Giro, Specialized, Vetta, Louis Garneau, Etto, LT, Monarch, Troxel, Trek Performance, and Schwinn are just a few of the brands you'll find on the market. Bell is the market leader. However, over the years I've conducted countless tests on helmets and can confidently say you have an excellent crop to pick from. Competition has forced manufacturers to remedy prickly problems such as strap and fastening systems. Most helmets weigh within a few grams of each other and offer similar amounts of cooling and air flow. Ultimately, your decision will likely be dictated by how the thing feels on your head. I try on most helmets and can't wear some, even those sized properly, because they don't fit my head well. In other words, they don't feel right. This is not the manufacturer's problem; the problem is with the weird shape of my head. I won't mention brands because it would be unfair to the manufacturers. I use those examples to underscore the importance of fit. If a helmet doesn't fit right, if it's parked on the back of the head like a straw hat, or moves around freely on your head, the helmet is of little use. The most common mistake for riders to make is to wear the helmet too far back, turning poor fit into a fashion statement. The helmet should be level in order to protect the frontal area of the brain. If it's too low, your vision will be impaired. A mirror will provide a quick check. Most helmets come with sizing pads that will allow you to form-fit a helmet to your head. Each helmet has a different retention system, so you should follow the accompanying instructions for strap adjustment. Just remember that the straps will lengthen owing to wear and weather and you'll be obliged to adjust them from time to time. Buckles are usually the "squeeze" or "snap" variety, with the latter being more common. It's simply easier to squeeze the buckle snap to unbuckle than to unsnap the buckle. Both straps and buckle should fit snugly but not tightly. In other words, the buckle shouldn't leave marks on your chin.

I recall participating in large-group bicycle rides and discovering by the 20-mile mark that many helmets were parked serenely on the rear racks or in the handlebar bags of the cyclists. Those were the days when helmets were too heavy and offered little ventilation. After a point, cyclists figured, safety be damned. My neck can't support the load any longer. Fortunately, helmet weight is no longer an excuse for not using the product and less likely to be the cause of neck pain. But neck pain is real enough and is still the bane of a lot of riders. Fortunately, you can do something about it.

REMEDIES

I know of participants in the arduous Race Across America who are unable to hold up their heads after the 2,000-mile mark. The reason is that the neck muscles are completely fatigued. Fortunately you're not likely to face such a serious problem. Neck strain and pain are not very common in mountain bikers because of their upright riding position. You're more likely to feel the twinge if you ride a road bike. But even here the pain can be significantly reduced or eliminated with attention to bike fit, riding position, and exercise.

If your stem is too long, the trapezius and other neck muscles will be strained because you are stretched out on the bike and obliged to bend the neck upward to get a good view of the road. The often-stated rule of thumb for stem length is that the handlebar should obscure the front hub when your hands are on the brake hoods. We spoke about proper setup for the mountain bike in Chapter 2. Ideally, you should make this determination when you are buying a bike, rather than waiting till you experience pain. If you want to purchase a particular bike and the stem seems too long, ask the salesperson to put on a shorter one. It's a minor adjustment. Or if you discover this after riding a few miles, return to the place of purchase. Most bike shops will make the change at little or no extra cost.

Conversely, if the hub is in front of the handlebar with you in the same position, you might need a longer stem, though that is far less typical. Many road riders like to feel and look long and stretched out on the bike and desire a longer stem than the body requires, often compensating for it by moving the saddle forward, which just creates another problem. Don't change the knee-over-the-pedal position discussed in Chapter 2.

Riding position and techniques can help reduce neck strain. Try not to hold your head in one position for a long period. When it's safe to do so, let your head drop to the chest and rotate it from side to side. You'll see cyclists frequently rubbing the back of their neck to reduce tension in the neck muscles. Be careful not to hunch your shoulders or hold the arms stiff because they transmit road shock to the neck. When riding conditions permit, stretch your arms and shoulders. Reach behind you with one arm, then the other. On a road with little or no traffic, I like to ride "no hands" so I can fully stretch my upper body and if necessary carefully massage my neck. Of course, you should practice this technique before trying it on the road. A bike that is in alignment should track straight. Riding "no hands" for a few seconds is a feat within everyone's capabilities.

Research shows that squinting in sunlight or hazy weather can significantly contribute to tension in the face and neck. So wear sunglasses even when it's not especially sunny. A model that blocks all ultraviolet light is your best choice. And get a model that doesn't slip down when you look down. Otherwise, the glasses can actually obscure your vision.

The aero handlebar, which many performance cyclists use to lower their profile and thereby reduce wind resistance, is another potential cause of neck strain. The bolt-on aero bar is a great addition to your arsenal if you are going to participate in time trials or triathlons. Fitness cyclists like the aero bar because it stretches them out and enables them to cover the same distance in less time. If you think an aero bar might be for you, here are some cautions: You'll likely need a new stem, as an aero bar changes your position and weight distribution on the bike. Get some advice from your local specialty shop. Then go slowly at first, giving your neck time to get used to it.

Off-bike exercises are an important regimen to help keep neck strain to a minimum. Stretch the neck muscles regularly. The simplest one involves bending the head to each side until the ear touches the shoulder and slowly rotating the head through its natural range of motion. In truth any stretching exercises that increase your overall flexibility will help reduce neck pain. The exercise options on Nautilus and similar equipment, including neck extension and tilts, are excellent ways to reduce neck strain. I've had far fewer neck problems since I've been using Nautilus equipment on a regular basis.

Even the most experienced riders feel some neck soreness in the early season as the muscles get used to holding up head and helmet. The soreness usually goes away after the first few rides. Don't forget to do basic stretches and neck rolls at rest stops. Consider them preventive maintenance.

Few cyclists I know have never experienced some kind of back pain. No wonder. Cycling puts a tremendous amount of pressure on our backs, which contribute to our cycling power, help even out our pedal cadence, and literally anchor us to the bike. The more aerodynamic we become on the bike, particularly when our hands are on the drops or we're using aero bars, the more stretched out we are and the more pressure the back feels. Add to this mix big gears, hill climbing, and washboard mountain bike terrain, and it's no wonder the back might howl on occasion.

Keep in mind our perspective. The bicycle is often prescribed for people with back problems. When I injured the L-5 disk in my lower back from falling on a hardwood floor, the pain down my leg was so intense I wanted to scream. A chiropractor didn't help. I got a second and third opinion and surgery was recommended. I saw the X rays and concurred but missed a return flight and had to cancel surgery. I figured that was an omen. With pain I climbed aboard my exercise bike. I could move no more than a fraction of an inch to either side.

To keep from moving my back, I put the bike between two support stanchions in the basement. Sometimes, I would hold them to relieve the pain while pedaling. After six months the pain subsided and eventually left. I had more X rays taken and these showed the area had healed itself.

Kathy Bambeck of Portland, Oregon, had a similar experience, suffering a pinched nerve in the back that caused pain in the legs and back. Her doctor sent her to a surgeon, who could not operate successfully on her back. Like most of us with pain, she began the free fall through specialists. Finally she stopped at a physical therapist who recommended the stationary bike for 30 minutes 3 days a week. Bored, she purchased a real bike and increased her mileage. The pain she suffered for twenty-five years is gone and doesn't return as long as she rides and does her other exercises. Her major goal is to cycle through Europe.

Russell Airbinder of Manorville, New York, was in an automobile accident that severely and permanently injured his back. He couldn't sit in a standard chair without discomfort, and at 6' 2" and 300 pounds, wasn't in shape to do other exercises. He learned about a recumbent bicycle, the kind you sit in like a lawn chair, and got one through his insurance. He is still in pain but gets around better without his cane and is cycling regularly. His blood pressure is lower and he finds it harder to get his heart into the training zone, a good sign.

Michael Motto of Kunkeltown, Pennsylvania, jumped on his mountain bike soon after disk surgery, and after riding some demanding single tracks, Michael was in so much pain that he thought he'd have to give up cycling completely. Not easily deterred, he decided to buy a mountain bike with suspension (shock absorbers) front and rear. He put on a slightly higher set of handlebars and limits his amount of "air time." He can now ride without pain. His weight has dropped from 224 pounds to 191 and he's dropped a full size in his clothes.

Santo Scolrao of Wahiawa, Hawaii, had a chronic back problem that contributed to the paralysis of his left leg. The doctor told him he had degenerative disk disease, and though the paralysis cleared, he would probably walk with a limp and a cane the rest of his life. His leg atrophied a half-inch.

Desperate, he looked to the bicycle for rehabilitation. His leg wasn't working, so he strapped it to the toe clip and dragged it around up to 10 miles, 4 days a week. The leg got stronger and the back pain lessened. After years of cycling, the pain has disappeared. Santo now lives without pain, cycling 120 miles a week to keep the disks in his back lubricated. He can do a century in 5 hours, a remarkable time. Remember, this is a man who was told he would walk with a limp and a cane the rest of his life.

I used these stories to put cycling backaches in perspective. Cycling heals rather than hurts the back. Any pain you might experience can be remedied through exercises and adjustment in your riding style. Research has shown that nearly 100 percent of the back injuries associated with cycling can be eliminated.

The best way to ward off and prevent backaches is to have strong abdominal muscles, advice that has broad application. During long rides the abdominal muscles tire and can't resist the pull of the back muscles. In this instance, the pelvis will rock from side to side as we cycle, eventually causing lower back muscles to fatigue. To strengthen back muscles, do "crunches" rather than traditional sit-ups, which have little effect on the abdominals. I do mine every morning after rolling out of bed, elevating my feet. I do at least 300 a day and can vouch for the efficacy of this exercise.

When looking for causes of back pain, look to bike fit, the principal offender. Usually the saddle is too high and the pelvis rocks from side to side, straining the back. The culprit could be fore and aft position of the saddle. Some racers move the saddle back as little as 2 centimeters to be in a position to push big gears. This can result in back problems. So can even slightly tilting the seat downward. Similarly, if the distance from handlebars to saddle is too far or too short, this could adversely affect the back.

If correct fit, riding position, and conditioning exercises don't alleviate a back problem on a road bike, by all means try a mountain or a cross bike. At the very least replace the drop handlebars with straight ones and consider putting on wider tires. There is evidence, though it's still spotty, that suspension systems could aggravate a back injury. The informed opinion from experienced mountain bikers is that rear suspension is good for lower back problems and front suspension for problems in the neck. But I don't offer that as medical advice. As in the examples cited above, experiment. See what works for you. Some people with back problems ride fully suspended bikes on pavement, thus assuring almost no jarring at all. Be careful and let your comfort level dictate your style of riding and terrain.

The next point of potential pain, endless contention, and a fair number of old wives' tales is the saddle, on which the most sensitive part of your anatomy perches. Thankfully the old days, when saddles were made primarily of leather and cyclists had to ride, beat, and oil them until they were "soft," are long gone. Saddles come in a dizzying array of shapes, sizes, and materials so that only the most sensitive plant won't find one that fits. Gel-filled saddles are very popular with recreational cyclists because they don't need breaking in. You can simply get on the bike and ride.

The saddles you find in any bike shop selection are there because some product manager decided they are what the customers want. Though there are many well-known, respected saddle manufacturers such as Selle Italia, Selle San Marco, Vetta, and Selle Royale, who produce their own labels plus saddles for Specialized, Avocet, and others, they don't have the notoriety that bike companies have. Too bad. Cycling on a comfortable saddle will contribute to your riding pleasure.

If you look at the underside of a saddle, you'll see two steel rails. Or two aluminum rails. Or two titanium rails. Plastic is customarily used as a foundation material. Padding is typically a foam or a gel. Cover material can be leather, nylon, suede, and Lycra. Since gel was introduced as the padding material almost twenty years ago, consumers have found saddles much more comfortable. Manufacturers have also responded to demands and created a variety of "anatomical" saddles that better suit the human anatomy, especially that of women. Beginners usually seek out a wide, soft saddle because, at first glance and on first ride, it seems comfortable. Performance riders want a narrower, firmer saddle with less flexibility because it enables them to deliver more power to the pedals. What you buy is a personal choice. If you plan to ride a mountain, cross, or road bike sitting in the upright position, a wider saddle would be fine. If you intend to race or train hard, you'll likely need a narrower saddle. Over a long ride a wide saddle will chafe the legs and cause discomfort. Contrary to conventional wisdom, having a lot of saddle padding does not decrease the friction in the area of the sit bones.

Men's sit bones are about $4\frac{1}{4}$ inches apart compared to $4\frac{3}{4}$ inches for women. For that reason, women's saddles are wide and slightly shorter than men's. That's the basic physiology. Finding the right saddle is often a matter of trial and error. Chances are the saddle that comes with the bike of your choice will suit you fine. If not, experiment. I do. I used a Selle Italia saddle for a few years, riding about 10,000 miles. Nothing fancy. It was a modified gel saddle on a plastic foundation with leather covering. The Selle Italia was my tweed jacket and Brittany spaniel. I took it everywhere in every weather. Then, two weeks before a ten-day European bike tour the plastic foundation cracked and the saddle leaned curiously to one side. Changing saddles is like changing partners; the process is often quite traumatic. The cracked saddle was no longer in production so in the days before my trip I tried to find a model with the same features. I probably road-tested a half-dozen saddles in one week, leading to a case of saddle sores. At the eleventh hour I decided to go with a Terry saddle with titanium rails. I liked the narrow nose of the saddle and figured the shape would favor my condition. Though the Terry got me through my long tour, it wasn't without some discomfort.

The moral is: Pay close attention to your saddle needs. After all, that's where your comfort sits. Don't rely too much on one saddle. Always have another one "broken in," ready to use. On a new saddle, figure your bottom will be a little sore after the first few rides but you will quickly toughen up. Unlike the traditional leather saddle that, after a "break-in" period, assumed the shape of one's anatomy, the gel saddles are not really broken in. You are, as the body gets used to the shape. The popular gel saddle provides firmness and support while taking some stress off the lower back.

Long-distance cyclists can get saddle sores, owing to long hours in the saddle. Personal hygiene, wearing clean bicycle shorts without underwear, sensible increases in ride duration and intensity, and rest days will take care of most problems. Because they are "out of the saddle" so much, mountain bikers rarely experience saddle soreness.

Any body point that contacts the bike is a potential source of discomfort, especially on a road bike. Most experienced cyclists have felt some discomfort or tingling in the hands during road shock, which compresses the ulnar nerve leading into the hands. Others report numbness and even nerve damage, though the latter is very rare. The popular name for damage to the ulnar nerve is handlebar palsy. All these conditions can be anticipated and remedied through proper bike position.

As you have learned in these pages, a saddle tilted down from the vertical will cause you to slide forward, thus putting pressure on the hands. A position that forces the elbows to be locked and hand grip tight on the handlebars will have the same effect. The key is to extend the notion of "soft riding" to how you actually hold the bike. Don't hang on for dear life, as many new cyclists do. Avoid any extended periods on the hooks of the drop handlebars. Rather, let the hands rest comfortably on the brake hoods. Keep moving your hands around. In truth, different road and weather conditions invite and encourage this movement anyway. By all means, use thickly padded gel gloves and padded handlebar tape.

For performance riders, use of an aero bar, which causes the weight to be carried on the forearm, eliminates any potential hand problems. Mountain bikers occasionally experience stress on the thumbs owing to the placement of the gear shift levers. This is usually remedied by moving the levers closer to the base of the thumb.

If cycling can occasionally be the cause of discomfort and degeneration, a state most often brought about by improper riding position, it's more often the cause of regeneration. We have seen examples of how cycling has brought an injured nerve to life. Earlier we learned the story of Austin Clark, who used cycling to help regenerate his injured nerve and soul. Then there was Tom Mueller, struck with Guillain-Barré syndrome, a nerve disorder that "short-circuited" his entire body. He came back to health, and along with good medical support, the bicycle was his vehicle. Robert Strickland of Boston, Massachusetts, was a high school quarterback and pole vaulter when he

191

was struck with a form of muscular dystrophy which affected the strength in his shoulders, arms, face, and chest muscles. He has lost much of his upper body strength, but the bike showed him he still has strength and speed in his legs. Cycling helped him regain his health and became a healing force in his life. Peter Bower, a cyclist, discovered he had a rare neurological disorder (chronic inflammatory demyelinating polyradiculoneuropathy) that caused numbness in his hands and feet. His blood was removed and filtered twice for six months. He was obliged to stay off the bike for fifteen months as the nerves grew back. When he returned to his sport with a mountain bike, he could go no farther than around the block. Now back on his road bike, he is able to again ride long distances. His feet are still numb and will be for the rest of his life, but his quadriceps are stronger than before. He has come back.

Most of the aches and pains associated with cycling are of no great importance. A little adjustment in riding style or equipment will take care of them. Cycling gives much more than it takes. To be fair, on-bike injuries are usually due to overtraining, a mistake in judgment rather than in activity. For example, the small number of cyclists who develop knee problems do so primarily because almost all push too big a gear or set the saddle too high.

Correct fit and technique would eliminate 80–90 percent of the problems. Remember, cycling is usually the first regimen recommended by many doctors and physical therapists after injury and surgery. The sport is safe, soft, and easy on the knees. True, anatomically variances do contribute to some knee problems but these tend to be the exceptions.

The most common knee problem associated with cycling is chondromalacia patellae, an irritation of cartilage under the kneecap. The pain is caused by friction of the kneecap on the thighbone. Again, though cycling can contribute to this condition, cycling can also remedy it. Though you should rely on formal medical diagnosis, you likely have chondromalacia if you hear a grinding or cracking in the knee when walking or bending. The pain will appear inside or on the underside of the knee after exercise.

As noted, bad bike fit can be a contributing factor, especially saddle height. So can a previous injury, genetics, and weak quads. More likely you've been overtraining, riding the hills too hard or too long, and pushing too big a gear, particularly before the body is ready. Treatment usually consists of icing and elevating the knee after riding, staying in low gears and out of the big chainring for a couple of months. Arthroscopic surgery might be necessary but only as a last resort. If you listen to your body early, you can probably anticipate and prevent this condition.

A less common knee problem is patella tendinitis at the kneecap or shinbone. Usually there is swelling and the tendon feels tender. You might experience this if one leg is longer than the other. More likely it's due to a low saddle and premature hard or hilly training. Ice will work here too, as well as aspirin or ibuprofen to reduce swelling. Long-term, adjust saddle height, find the low gears, and take rest days seriously. If you have a leg length discrepancy, an orthotic might be in order.

Between 10 and 15 percent of all cycling injuries are due to tendinitis in the quadriceps, an inflammation where this tendon passes over the kneecap. You notice swelling and discomfiture a few inches above the knee cap. Heavy off-season weight training can exacerbate this condition, usually caused by improper saddle height and big gear cycling. You're vulnerable to this complaint if you increase your mileage too quickly.

Illiotibial band syndrome, an irritation of the tendon on the outside of the thigh and marked by a sharp pain on the thighbone, may be due to bowed legs, wide hips, or pointing the toes in toward the bike while pedaling. Fixed clipless pedals can also contribute to this condition. More attention to fit, especially seat height, might help as well as the use of what's called "floating" clipless pedals, which I'll discuss shortly.

There are a few other knee conditions such as a strain of the hamstring tendon and most are due to human error, not anatomy, though you'll have to take your genetics into consideration. Flat feet and leg-length discrepancy can contribute to knee problems. More likely they are due to low saddle and low pedal cadence. The remedies should be obvious by now. Similarly, mistakes we all make in our training can be the culprit too. As I've discussed, one has the tendency to push hard early in the season because the bike is seductive. I've reiterated the need for low-gear, foundation mileage. That alone will help prevent many knee problems. So will keeping the knees warm, especially below 55°F.

Cycling footwear has undergone significant changes in the last ten years. Before that a cyclist had two choices. The first was a cycling shoe with a soft top and hard shank and grooves on the sole to help keep the foot from moving. With a touring or fitness riding shoe, the feet weren't fixed on the pedal cage. The primary advantage of these shoes was they provided a stiff shank that had contact with the cage. These shoes are still available and popular with recreational cyclists. More rugged mountain bike models have become very popular. The other option was usually a European-made shoe, with a leather upper, which allowed the foot to "breathe," and a hard shank which accepted a cleat that attached to the pedal. The shoe was held in place by toe clips and straps, never a fully satisfactory arrangement. Toe clips and straps, though still seen on the road, are considered outdated technology, replaced by various pedal systems (Look, Time, Shimano, and others that actually clip on to the pedals, holding the foot much more securely than the toe clips, straps, and cleats). I was one of the last holdouts on the *Bicycling* staff to go with this new technology and now wonder why I waited so long. Gone is the occasional numbness felt in my feet on long rides. Gone is the reduced circulation in my feet from tightening the strap too tight in search of the phantom speed. Gone are the times I inadvertently pulled the pedal out of the clip. Gone are the days my feet move around too much on the pedal cage. So, for the performance rider, I absolutely endorse what is called a "clipless pedal" system. Easy to get in and out of, these pedals will definitely improve your cycling. Cyclists who ski will feel right at home with clipless pedal systems because they, too, have a spring-loaded release mechanism that is easy to exit, especially in an emergency. Beginners often fear being anchored too permanently to the pedals. Fear not. Turn the foot slightly to the right or left or some variation, depending on the model, and you will be free. I've only fallen once at a red light because I was not paying attention. You'll deliver more power to the pedals and make a reality all the advice about pedaling in the "round." At least you'll be able to do a fair imitation of pulling up on the pedal, thus evening out your stroke.

There is a biomechanical consideration for cyclists who adopt a clipless system. Though most cyclists will be well served by the standard systems on the market, some have experienced pain because the foot is more precisely fixed than with the traditional toe clips and straps, which permit a degree of lateral movement. The clipless system is designed to lock the foot securely in place and does its job well. One apparent result, however, is an increase in cyclists reporting some of the knee problems discussed above, including tendinitis and chondromalacia. Peter Francis, Ph.D., a mechanical engineer very familiar with clipless systems, suggests most cyclists can ride comfortably with the play provided by conventional clipless systems. For those who feel they need more play owing to injury or biomechanic imbalance, manufacturers have responded by designing clipless pedals that permit the foot to "float" or move laterally up to 10 degrees or more without any significant loss of power. For that reason alone, cyclists with a history of knee problems might want to consider using Look, Time, or other systems that offer this feature.

Be careful of diagnosing your real or imagined biomechanical irregularities yourself. Chances are you can use a traditional or floating clipless system from day one without adverse effects, assuming you go easy and let your ankles and knees grow used to the stresses and torques. But if you have severe knee problems or other biomechanical irregularities, you might want to chat with someone knowledgeable about the finer points of bike fit. A bike shop is a place to start. These days many have access to professional fit systems such as FitKit, which renders precise measurements. Occasionally you are lucky enough to have a trainer at a local health club who understands the biomechanics of cycling. Cyclists in the Denver area have access to Western Orthopedic Sports Medicine & Rehabilitation and the services of Andrew Pruitt, Ed.D. Pruitt, who works with the elite riders at the Olympic Training Center in Colorado Springs, is one of the most knowledgeable cycling trainers in the country and is a prototype for what the rest of the nation needs. He uses computer analysis to analyze pedal stroke and riding position. Most of us won't need this level of analysis, but if you do, find a trainer or sports medicine doctor who knows something about cycling. They are becoming easier to find by the day.

Ultimately, your footwear will depend on the type of riding you do. I still see plenty of tourists who are quite happy with traditional touring shoes. However, if performance is your game, you'll want to give serious consideration to the clipless systems that can be used on road and mountain bikes, though a heavier, thicker version of the touring shoe is popular with recreational mountain bikers. Clipless systems are not inexpensive, ranging in price from $65 to $180 for shoes and cleats. But neither are running shoes that cost about the same.

Feeling one with the bike presupposes you can cycle without discomfort and pain. That countless athletes and nonathletes use the bike to reduce pain and come back from the most traumatic injuries is sufficient evidence that, when used right, the bike will do no damage to the body. Unlike some of its sister sports, cycling does not need to issue a yearly calendar of pain. Cycling is the release, not the cause.

Cycling is the ideal health and fitness activity because you can do it all year and for a lifetime. In any weather and in any state of decay. The sport has its seasons and tributaries. One day this bike, the other day that. The surface changes. The hills are meaner or more hospitable. We dream endlessly of France. Goals appear in the spring like a blessing. New technology taunts us with the threat of getting better. The sport offers enough for every taste. We have seen the injured crawling around the neighborhood on a recumbent and speedster who finds 35 mph on his cyclometer. Both are welcome under this large health and fitness tent. Both cycle for fundamentally the same reason. To find health, to discover life. One crawls, the other flies. They both hear the same raucous music of mobility. No one that has heard the bike sing relegates the activity to a corner closet. Rather, cycling is the central flywheel around which much of life turns, especially for those who have suffered from being able to turn too little. I'm hesitant to claim that cycling is more than a sum of the parts, the collection of bike and rider, but my experience and intuition keep evoking metaphors rather than miles. With scuba diving the first thrill is to learn to dive with a breathing apparatus. After that the thrill is diving almost "breathlessly" through the beautiful waters, disturbing nothing but seeing it all. That has been my experience. I feel the same way about cycling. The bike, skills, and stuff are what you pick up on the way to the train station where the journey really begins. You might be fleet-footed and get to the station well in advance of departure time. Or you might be hobbling, walking with a cane, or dragging a damaged limb behind. You don't look as smart as the earlier arrival when climbing aboard, but once there, you are both equal, brothers in the saddle, joined democratically at the hip by the gearing. The equality is not always in the speed but in the potential. To move at all when movement was previously denied is a victory of no small consequence.

Let the nuts and bolts of the sport enter you as you enter a dream. Know them well, plaster them on your handlebars, recite the formulas like prayers. Then taste the hum of cycling. Let it take you back to your youth, forward to your promise, inside like a heartbeat. Push some more. Earn all the health and fitness awards that your phantom doctor offers. Push some more. Find speed and conquer it. Find power and conquer it. Then find companionship, serenity, and peace, and savor these rewards that come to those who cycle through the blue waters, barely making a sound.

Congratulations. You are indeed one with the bike.

C·H·A·P·T·E·R T·H·I·R·T·E·E·N

REGENERATION

The end is the beginning. The journey is cyclical but moves you forward nonetheless, if only incrementally. The shortest distance between two points grows as the world bends on its axis. I want to go due west, but as I discovered in the Navy, the magnetic compass throws the poles into confusion. I want to go this way and that. Sometimes I don't know what end's up. The ridge line falls toward me and I must demure. The single track offers a thick patch of primeval forest and I must linger. The hills point a finger and the weather obliges. I get sidetracked. Along the way, I truly celebrate the Olympians and coaches who have defined the artistry of our sport but find myself in the byways, shouting encouragement to those who can hardly walk. I look in vain for the parade of medical specialists who will underscore my anecdotes with full authority but am disappointed. I return to the baseline and trumpet the advice that will start the wheels turning. I celebrate the bike in all its elegance and simplicity but look constantly for the driver, he or she who rises from the ashes. I take you through the hills and dales, the traffic, the hazardous single track, and declare you saved and whole. When you feel safe, I give you other things to wear. I resist being the huckster. I want the activity to remain clean. But I run up your costs. I say "you decide," then invest chapters in persuading you. I itch to transcend the technical talk but want to make sure your hands are greasy. I tell you that cycling is almost too simple for words but stutter, lose my step, and complicate things. I have taken you for a ride.

I trust it's been an enjoyable one. There are enough fine books on the market that triumphantly carve a bike into its requisite bits, announcing in grim statistics that the beast has more than a thousand parts. I can't do that half as well. One reason I wrote this book is I got weary of hearing that the primary reason for cycling was "to feel the wind in one's hair," which to me was like equating sex with heavy breathing. You mean, that's all there is? Technology fuels this game and does so beautifully; without the advances of the last ten years we might be looking at a 2×4 on wheels, an archaic cadaver. Thank goodness for lightness, gears that click instead of rage, and bodies that melt over bikes like butter. Thank goodness for the mountain bike that celebrates our untutored genius. I love it. I particularly love the accoutrements of speed such as aero bars, bullet helmets, and one-piece Lycra suits that can occasionally allow us to slip inside the west wind. The poet Shelley would be pleased. But for every mile we gain, we give hope to those whose life is a game of inches. Every time I snap into my fine clipless pedals, I think of my fellow cyclist who tapes one leg to the pedal cage, hoping in time the leg will remember motion and the nerves will grow like the rivers the road is meant to be. When I complain of saddle discomfort, I think of Steve Rodnar of Madison, Wisconsin, who had most of his colon removed except the part that sits on the bicycle seat. The surgery went smoothly but soon he had to face the deaths of a favorite aunt, an army buddy who committed suicide, and his sister's husband, who was killed in a car crash. He wanted to die but he didn't. Steve got back on his bike and progressed until he was able to do a century. In his words, "Without my bike I would not have survived."

Lloyd R. Mackey of Ottawa, Ontario, suffers from Crohn's disease, a condition that causes inflammation and ulceration of the bowels. Fortunately his cycling has kept the disease under control with minimal medication, a rarity according to his physician. Can a doctor put a condition any more succinctly than this man? "I cycle 90 miles a week, from May to October, and in the winter train on a set of rollers and also speed-skate. The mileage may not seem significant but I find it necessary to listen to my body and have plenty of rest in order not to push myself too much. I feel there are four aspects to cycling and physical fitness that are significant benefactors to people with chronic conditions. First, physical fitness means a stronger body and constitution. This means the body is able to fight off a disease. Second, with my interest in fitness I eat nutritional food that benefits my cycling and keeps the disease under control. Third, cycling relieves stress, which can cause a condition to worsen. Four, physical activity produces endorphins as a natural regenerative process. This continued production of natural healing agents could also provide a healing activity in the affected areas of the bowel. Now these premises are not substantiated by the medical profession and I don't know if there is any validity to them. I only know since I have taken up cycling, my condition has improved and I've never felt better."

Actually, the medical profession would support all or most of these points. More important, perhaps, is that Mackey has taken such an interest in his health and healing. If he has not become his own doctor, he has become the agent of healing. He has recognized that he has the power within to significantly improve his life. If he can, we can too.

We live and grow by example, analogy, and decay. Our life quickens when we learn of a death, our resolve hardens when we witness the anguish of immobility. William H. Richardson of Indianapolis was told by his surgeon, after a high-speed motorcycle accident, that he would never walk again without a cane. He would certainly have arthritis. Three months after the accident he rented a stationary bike, strapped the bad foot to the pedal and cycled. The pain was so severe he felt faint and often cried. He persevered, and after four months was able to complete a full circle. Soon he was on a used ten-speed, then a Schwinn, Cannondale, and Diamondback mountain bike. He races seriously. Bill Richardson concludes: "I do not now or ever have since the accident walked with a cane."

This example represents a regeneration of body and spirit. Bill's health is better as is his outlook on life. He had brought his wife to cycling. And all this started with him shattered in a cornfield on his way to an eight-hour operation to repair, among other things, his right femur, which looked like an open flower.

Paul Swift of Kenosha, Illinois, became ill with Kawasaki disease, which attacks the lymph glands and important organs. He thought he would never cycle again and his doctor offered little promise. The comeback is similar. First a walk to the end of the block, then a short bike ride. The world opened up and his condition improved. But Paul Swift didn't stop there. He is a five-time national cycling champion and has been a member of the United States cycling team for ten years. I have seen this man race at the Lehigh County Velodrome not far from my office. He is a powerful, determined athlete who knows something about transcendence.

What is it about cycling that so attracts the charities? The Lung Association, the Heart Association, Muscular Dystrophy, and Multiple Sclerosis all use bike events to raise funds. MS has been very successful, raising a high percentage of its operating funds through cycling, a fund raiser even more popular than the ugly bartender contest, cycling's equivalent of the decidedly politically incorrect dwarf toss. The events are sometimes half-ghoulishly referred to as the "disease rides" and they are that. But if disease is the organizing principle, health is the objective. I've often wondered why cyclists coming to health and fitness often use an MS ride as a rite of passage, their coming out. The events are handy, of course, occurring in a hundred neighborhoods, and that helps. The events are well managed and that helps too. My guess is the primary reason so many up-and-coming cyclists use these events is to give something back. We all skate on the edge of disease and unhealth, and those who have been on the other side understand how precious a gift health is. For others, cycling permits them nothing more than an opportunity to stay on the edge of pain, enjoying life to the fullest. A recreational cyclist from Park Forest, Illinois, who asked me not to use his name for fear of losing his Social Security disability benefits, suffers rheumatoid arthritis in his hands, wrists, elbows, shoulders, the right side of his jaw, hips, knees, ankles, and feet. To combat the pain and reduce the swelling, he's taking a steroid, an anti-inflammatory drug, and methotrexate, used for transplant patients. They don't work very well. To escape the wheelchair, he started cycling, using Scott clip-on aero bars to take pressure off his hands and wrists. He now rides more than 3,000 miles a year. He is still in pain and likely always will be but he can forget about his disability when he rides, cruising the country lanes at 20 mph.

Valerie Larson of Seattle notes, "I won't be the fastest on the course, but I'm on the course and that's really what counts." This book has been about that meandering course through bike parts, training regimens, and success stories. Flannery O'Connor, a favorite author of mine, said sometimes you have to draw large and startling figures to get people's attention. She was talking about religion, not cycling, but maybe there's a connection. With the help of so many generous people who have unselfishly and candidly relayed their stories to me, I hope I've been able to provide a human backdrop against which your cycling accomplishments can be measured. Moreover, I hope these stories have inspired you as much as they have inspired me.

This book is about action. I want you to get out and ride. That's the most important decision; the others will come as you embrace the sport. Wherever you are, no matter the state of your health, cycling will meet you there. Give it time and cycling will lead you to health. Moreover, the sport can regenerate body and soul.

This story ends but your story begins. The end is the beginning. My effort is really not complete until I hear from you. I want to learn about your comeback to health. Tell me your bike-centered tales of woe and regeneration. Talk to me about your "inner game of cycling."

I can be reached at *Mountain Bike* magazine, 33 East Minor Street, Emmaus, Pennsylvania 18098.

Appendixes

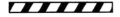

APPENDIX A

Frame Sizes

50 cm = 19.7 in.
51 cm = 20.1 in.
52 cm = 20.5 in.
53 cm = 20.9 in.
54 cm = 21.3 in.
55 cm = 21.7 in.
56 cm = 22.0 in.
57 cm = 22.4 in.
58 cm = 22.8 in.
59 cm = 23.2 in.
60 cm = 23.6 in.
61 cm = 24.0 in.
62 cm = 24.4 in.
63 cm = 24.8 in.
64 cm = 25.2 in.
65 cm = 25.6 in.

Note whether the measurement is from the center of the bottom bracket to the center or top of the top tube. A frame measuring 56 cm center-to-center is nearly 1 cm larger than one measuring 56 cm center-to-top.

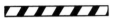

APPENDIX B

Bike Fit

Inseam (cm) × 0.65 = frame size (cm, center-to-center)
Inseam (cm) × 0.883 = saddle height (cm, from center of bottom bracket to top of saddle)

(Measure your inseam, in bare feet, from floor to crotch.)

Inseam (cm)	Crank arm length (mm)	Measured from the center of the bottom bracket axle to the center of the pedal mounting hole. Crank arm length is usually marked on the back of the arm.
Less than 74	165	
74–80	170	
81–86	172.5	
87–93	175	

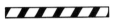

APPENDIX C

Gearing

$$\text{Gear inches} = \frac{\text{Wheel diameter (26 or 27 inches)} \times \text{chainring teeth}}{\text{cog teeth}}$$

Use 27 inches for 700C wheels. A common misconception is that gear inches equal the distance traveled in one crankarm revolution. Not so. To get that figure, multiply gear inches by pi (3.14).

A gear chart calculates inches for every usable cog and chainring combination. Tape a copy to the top of your stem to help you learn the location of the next higher or lower gear.

	42	53
13	×	110
14	81	102
15	76	95
16	71	89
17	67	84
19	60	75
21	54	×

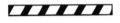

APPENDIX D

Heart Rate Formulas

Approximate maximum = 220 − age

Approximate training target
    Lower limit = 0.6 × maximum heart rate
    Upper limit = 0.8 × maximum heart rate

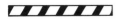

APPENDIX E

Training Programs

Goal: To Ride 100 Miles

Week	Mon. Easy	Tues. Pace	Wed. Brisk	Thur.	Fri. Pace	Sat. Pace	Sun. Pace	Total Weekly Mileage
1.	6	10	12	Off	10	30	9	77
2.	7	11	13	Off	13	34	10	86
3.	8	13	15	Off	13	38	11	98
4.	8	14	17	Off	14	42	13	108
5.	9	15	19	Off	15	47	14	119
6.	11	15	21	Off	15	53	16	131
7.	12	15	24	Off	15	59	18	143
8.	13	15	25	Off	15	65	20	153
9.	15	15	25	Off	15	65	20	155
10.	15	15	25	Off	10	5 Easy	Century	170

Goal: A Century with Strength to Spare

Week	Mon. Easy	Tues. Pace	Wed. Brisk	Thur.	Fri. Pace	Sat. Pace	Sun. Pace	Total Weekly Mileage
1.	10	12	14	Off	12	40	15	103
2.	10	13	15	Off	13	44	17	112
3.	10	15	17	Off	15	48	18	123
4.	11	16	19	Off	16	53	20	135
5.	12	18	20	Off	18	59	22	149
6.	13	19	23	Off	19	64	24	162
7.	14	20	25	Off	20	71	27	177
8.	16	20	27	Off	20	75	29	187
9.	17	20	30	Off	20	75	32	192
10.	19	20	30	Off	10	5 Easy	Century	184

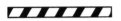

APPENDIX F

Shoes

Fore/Aft Position (conventional cleats)

Shoe Size	39	40	41	42	43	44	45	46	47
Distance (cm)	10.6	11	11.4	11.8	12.2	12.6	13	13.4	13.8

Measured from the center of the cleat slot to the front of the sole.

Fore/Aft Position (lock cleats)

Shoe Size	39	40	41	42	43	44	45	46	47
Distance (cm)	7.9	8.3	8.7	9.1	9.5	9.9	10.3	10.7	11.1

Draw a line on the sole that corresponds to the given distance. Position the cleat so this line is over the center of the pedal axle.

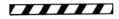

APPENDIX G

Speed

$$\text{Current speed (mph)} = \frac{(\text{gear inches} \times 3.14) \times (\text{rpm} \times 60)}{63{,}360}$$

$$\text{Average speed} = \frac{\text{distance traveled (miles)}}{\text{time (hours)}}$$

To convert minutes to fractions of an hour, divide by 60.

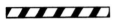

APPENDIX H

Menus
_____

Day 1

Breakfast	Serving Size	Calories	Fat (g)
Cranberry juice	4 oz.	65	<1
Bagel	1	163	1
Cream cheese, light	1 oz.	74	7
Fruited low-fat yogurt	½ cup	115	1
Lunch			
Sandwich			
Whole wheat bread	2 slices	123	2
Ham (extra lean)	1 oz.	38	1
Mozzarella cheese (part skim)	1 oz.	72	5
Mayonnaise (light)	1 tbsp.	40	4
Lettuce, romaine	¼ cup	2	<1
Tomato	¼	6	<1
Minestrone soup	1 cup	86	3
Apple	1	81	<1
Water			

Snack

Banana	1	105	<1
Skim milk	1 cup	86	<1

Dinner

Tossed salad	1 cup	31	<1
Italian dressing (low cal.)	2 tbsp.	31	3
Chicken breast (no skin, roasted)	3 oz.	140	3
Broccoli, cooked	½ cup	26	<1
Margarine, diet	1 tsp.	17	2
Potato, baked	1	115	<1
Sour cream, light	2 tbsp.	59	6
Italian bread	2 slices	170	0
Coffee	1 cup	5	0
Pear	1	97	<1
Water			

Snack

Rice pudding (with 2% milk)	1 cup	320	5
Water			

Total Calories 2,067
Total Fat. . . . . 45 grams
Percent of Calories from Fat 19%
Dietary Fiber . . . . 30 grams

Day 2

Breakfast	Serving Size	Calories	Fat (g)
Orange juice	½ cup	56	<1
Raisin bran	1 cup	154	1
Skim milk	½ cup	43	<1
Banana	1	105	<1
Coffee	1 cup	56	0

Lunch

Cheese enchilada (commercial)	1	320	19
Cooked rice	1 cup	264	<1
Tossed salad	1 serving	32	<1
Salad dressing (low-fat)	2 tbsp.	32	3
Melon wedges	1 cup	56	<1
Water			

Snack

Pretzel	1	60	1
Chocolate pudding (low-fat)	¹/₂ cup	193	6
Water			

Dinner

Flounder	3 oz.	100	1
Squash puree	¹/₂ cup	58	1
Fresh romaine, tomato, and onion	1 cup	59	1
Hard rolls	2	205	2
Butter	1 tsp.	36	4
Fruit salad	1 cup	125	<1
Water			

Snack

Monterey jack cheese (low-fat)	1 oz.	79	6
Crackers, Triscuits	5	105	4
Water			

Total Calories 2,087
Total Fat. . . . . 50 grams
Percent of Calories from Fat 21%
Dietary Fiber . . . . 27 grams

Day 3

Breakfast	Serving Size	Calories	Fat (g)
Grape juice	4 oz.	58	<1
Blueberry muffin	1	110	4
Shredded wheat	1	83	<1
Raisins	1/4 cup	109	<1
Skim milk	1/2 cup	43	<1
Coffee	1 cup	5	0
Lunch			
Vegetable beef soup	1 cup	75	2
Spinach/mushroom salad	1 1/4 cups	20	<1
Oil/vinegar dressing	2 tbsp.	140	16
Swiss cheese and tomato sandwich			
Cracked wheat bread	2 slices	131	2
Low-fat Swiss cheese	1 oz.	97	7
Tomato slices	2	6	<1
Milk (1%)	1 cup	102	3
Snack			
Yogurt (low-fat, fruit-flavored)	1/2 cup	115	1
Banana	1	105	<1
Water			
Dinner			
Stir-fried chicken	2 oz.	86	2
and vegetables	2 cups	216	<1
Lo mein noodles	2 cups	366	2
Water			
Orange	1	62	<1

Snack

English muffin	1	154	1
Jam	1 tbsp.	55	0
Herb tea	1 cup	2	0

Total Calories 2,140
Total Fat. . . . . 41 grams
Percent of Calories from Fat 17%
Dietary Fiber . . . . 30 grams

Day 4

Breakfast	Serving Size	Calories	Fat (g)
Grapefruit	1/2	37	<1
Cooked oatmeal	1 cup	145	2
Milk (1%)	1/2 cup	51	1
Toasted raisin bread	1 slice	70	1
Coffee	1 cup	5	0

Lunch			
Baked potato	1	220	<1
Chili con carne topping	3/4 cup	255	12
Tossed salad	6 oz.	32	<1
Vinaigrette dressing			
Olive oil	2 tsp.	80	9
Vinegar	1 tbsp.		

Snack			
Pear	1	98	<1
Water			

Dinner			
Lasagna (vegetable)	6 oz.	240	14
Cucumber salad with onions and yogurt	1/2 cup	53	1
Italian bread	2 slices	170	0
Raspberries	1/2 cup	30	<1
Yogurt	4 oz.	100	2

Snack

Fig bars	2 oz.	318	6
Herb tea	1 cup	2	0

Total Calories 1,906
Total Fat. . . . . 49 grams
Percent of Calories from Fat 23%
Dietary Fiber . . . . 28 grams

Day 5

Breakfast	Serving Size	Calories	Fat (g)
Apricot nectar	6 oz.	96	<1
Scrambled egg	1	101	8
Corn bread	1 serving	120	2
Apple butter	2 tbsp.	74	<1
Herb tea	8 oz.	2	0
Lunch			
Split pea soup	1 cup	188	4
Salad: broccoli, cauliflower, radishes, & lettuce	2 cups	37	<1
Salad dressing, ranch	2 tbsp.	60	6
Pita	1	105	1
Water			
Snack			
Gingersnap cookies	4	138	7
Banana	1	105	<1
Water			
Dinner			
Spinach pasta topped with	4 oz.	147	1
marinara sauce	1 cup	170	8
olive oil	2 tsp.	80	9
Steamed zucchini	1/3 cup	12	<1

Italian bread	2 slices	170	0
Blueberries with	½ cup	41	<1
non-fat yogurt	1 cup	127	<1
Water			

Snack

| Apple | 1 | 81 | <1 |

Total Calories 1,854
Total Fat. . . . . 48 grams
Percent of Calories from Fat 23%
Dietary Fiber . . . . 22 grams

Day 6

Breakfast	Serving Size	Calories	Fat (g)
Orange	1	62	<1
Non-fat yogurt	1 cup	127	<1
Granola	½ cup	297	17
Tea	1 cup	2	0

Lunch

Pizza	2 slices	280	6
Tossed green salad	2 cups	64	<1
Dressing	2 tbsp.	48	3
Cola	8 oz.	101	0

Snack

| Banana | 1 | 105 | <1 |
| Water | | | |

Dinner

Beef pot pie	5 oz.	348	20
Corn on the cob	1 ear	83	1
Spinach	½ cup	11	<1
Italian bread	2 slices	170	0
Grapes	1 serving	114	1
Tea	1 cup	0	0

Snack
Popcorn (plain)	3 cups	75	0
Water			

Total Calories 1,887
Total Fat . . . . 50 grams
Percent of Calories from Fat 23%
Dietary Fiber . . . . 33 grams

Day 7

Breakfast	Serving Size	Calories	Fat (g)
Cheerios with	1¹/₂ cups	133	2
Strawberries	¹/₂ cup	22	<1
Skim milk	¹/₂ cup	43	<1
Wheat toast	2 slices	135	2
Jam	2 tbsp.	110	0
Tea	1 cup	2	0
Lunch			
Chicken noodle soup	1 cup	75	3
Turkey sandwich	2 oz.	89	2
Cracked wheat bread	2 slices	130	2
Lettuce	2 leaves	5	<1
Mustard	1 tsp.	4	<1
Coleslaw with oil and vinegar	¹/₂ cup	88	7
Water			
Snack			
Graham crackers	2	60	2
Peanut butter	1 tbsp.	94	8
Peach	1	37	<1
Dinner			
Veal parmigiana (frozen entree)	5 oz.	197	9
Broccoli	1 cup	44	<1

Italian bread	2 slices	170	0
Cooked barley with	1 cup	193	<1
mushrooms	1/2 cup	9	<1
onions	1/2 cup	30	<1
olive oil	1 tsp.	40	5
Water			

Snack

Tangerine	1	36	<1
Almonds	1 tbsp.	48	4
Non-fat yogurt	1/2 cup	64	<1
Hummus	1/4 cup	105	5
Pita	1	105	<1
Tea	1 cup	2	0

Total Calories 2,077
Total Fat. . . . . 53 grams
Percent of Calories from Fat 22%
Dietary Fiber . . . . 38 grams

Courtesy of Anita Hirsch

Illustrations

BAR END SHIFTER

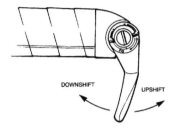

DOWNSHIFT   UPSHIFT

CLIPLESS PEDAL ENGAGEMENT

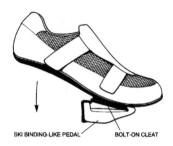

SKI BINDING-LIKE PEDAL   BOLT-ON CLEAT

CORNERING

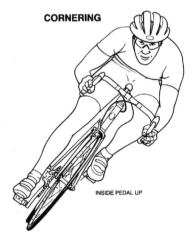

INSIDE PEDAL UP

HELMET ADJUSTMENT

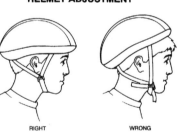

RIGHT   WRONG

RAPID FIRE SHIFTERS

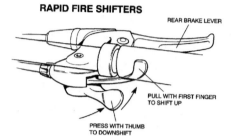

REAR BRAKE LEVER

PULL WITH FIRST FINGER
TO SHIFT UP

PRESS WITH THUMB
TO DOWNSHIFT

GRIP SHIFT

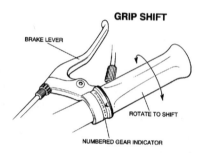

BRAKE LEVER

ROTATE TO SHIFT

NUMBERED GEAR INDICATOR

DUAL CONTROL LEVER

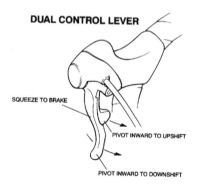

SQUEEZE TO BRAKE

PIVOT INWARD TO UPSHIFT

PIVOT INWARD TO DOWNSHIFT

HYBRID/CROSS BIKE

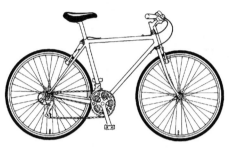

FRONT SUSPENSION

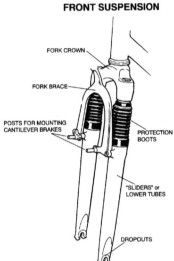

FORK CROWN

FORK BRACE

POSTS FOR MOUNTING
CANTILEVER BRAKES

PROTECTION
BOOTS

"SLIDERS" or
LOWER TUBES

DROPOUTS

TIRE COMPARISON

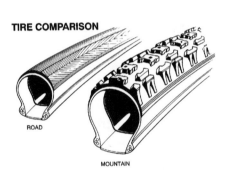

ROAD

MOUNTAIN

STEMS

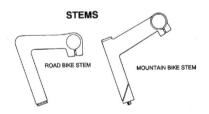

ROAD BIKE STEM

MOUNTAIN BIKE STEM

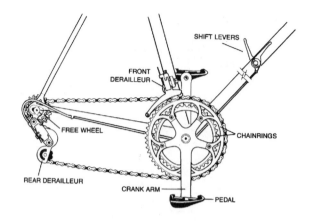

SHIFT LEVERS

FRONT DERAILLEUR

CHAINRINGS

FREE WHEEL

REAR DERAILLEUR

CRANK ARM

PEDAL

THE DRIVE TRAIN

FRAME GEOMETRY

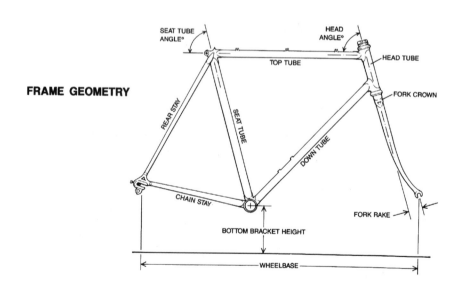

SEAT TUBE ANGLE°

HEAD ANGLE°

HEAD TUBE

TOP TUBE

REAR STAY

SEAT TUBE

DOWN TUBE

FORK CROWN

CHAIN STAY

FORK RAKE

BOTTOM BRACKET HEIGHT

WHEELBASE

SIZING COMPONENTS

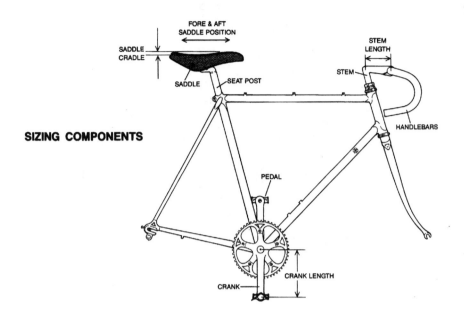

FORE & AFT
SADDLE POSITION

SADDLE
CRADLE

SADDLE

SEAT POST

STEM
LENGTH

STEM

HANDLEBARS

PEDAL

CRANK LENGTH

CRANK

CLINCHERS AND TUBULARS

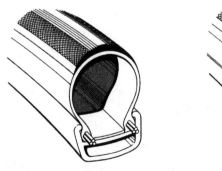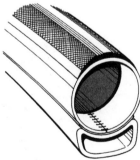

CLINCHER

TUBULAR

ROAD/SPORT BIKE

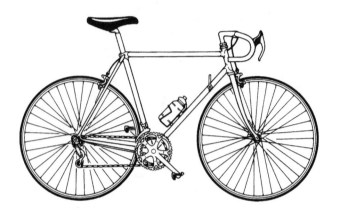

MOUNTAIN BIKE

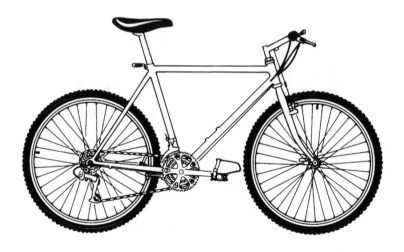

I·N·D·E·X

WIN A 1-YEAR SUBSCRIPTION TO

Mountain BIKE

MAGAZINE!

One-hundred lucky winners nationwide will receive a free one-year subscription to *Mountain Bike*, the ultimate mountain biking magazine. Find out about the latest trails, the coolest rides, the hottest new bike brands, and much, much more!

To enter, complete the coupon below and return to:

Cycling for Health, Fitness, and Well-Being Drawing
DTP Trade Paperbacks, Bantam Doubleday Dell Publishing Group, Inc.
Dept IR, 1540 Broadway, New York, NY 10036

ALL ENTRIES MUST BE RECEIVED BY JUNE 15, 1995

Please print the following information:

Name:

Address:

City: State: Zip:

Telephone: Age:

No purchase necessary. See Official Rules on back for details.

DTP
Trade Paperbacks

Sweepstakes Official Rules

1. NO PURCHASE NECESSARY. Enter by completing the Entry Coupon and return- ing it to the address provided or print your name, address, age and phone num- ber on a 3 x 5 card and send it to Cycling for Health, Fitness and Well-Being Drawing, DTP Trade Paperbacks, Bantam Doubleday Dell Publishing Group, Inc., Dept. IR, 1540 Broadway, New York, NY 10036. Only one entry per person allowed.

2. All entries must be received by DTP Trade Paperbacks no later than June 15, 1995. BDD is not responsible for late, lost or misdirected entries, and all entries become the property of BDD and will not be returned. Incomplete or illegible entries will not be accepted. Winners will be chosen in a random drawing on or about July 1, 1995 from among all completed entries received and will be noti- fied by mail. BDD's decision is final. Odds of winning are determined by the number of entries received.

3. One-hundred winners. One prize as follows: A one-year subscription to *Mountain Bike* magazine. Approximate value of prize is $17.00. No prize substi- tution or transfer allowed. Winners may be required to execute and return within 14 days of notification an affidavit of eligibility and release. In the event of non- compliance with this time period, an alternate winner will be chosen. If a winner is a minor the prize may be awarded in the parent's name.

4. This sweepstakes is open to residents of the U.S. and Canada, who are at least 13 years old at the time of entry. Employees of BDD and *Mountain Bike* magazine and their immediate family members are not eligible. The winner, if Canadian, will be required to answer correctly, a time-limited arithmetical skill-testing ques- tion in order to be awarded the prize. All federal, state and local rules apply. Void where prohibited or restricted by law. Taxes, if any, are the sole responsibili- ty of the winner. If legally permissible in the applicable state, entering the sweepstakes constitutes permission for the use of the winners' name and likeness for advertising and promotional purposes with no additional compensation.

5. For a list of winners, send a stamped, self-addressed envelope, entirely separate from your entry, by August 15, 1995 to: Cycling for Health, Fitness, and Well- Being magazine offer, DTP Trade Paperbacks, Dept IR, 1540 Broadway, New York, NY 10036.

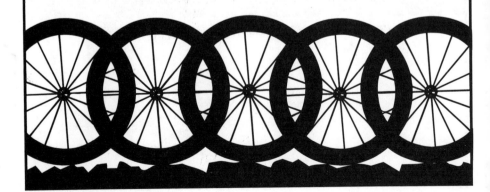